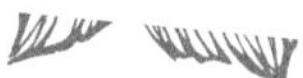

All right, Green Smoothie time!

Cleanse your body with Detox Diet and

Lose Up to 25 Pounds in 50 Days!

50 Days DETOX Diet Plan

with 50 Delicious Quick & Easy Green Smoothie Recipes

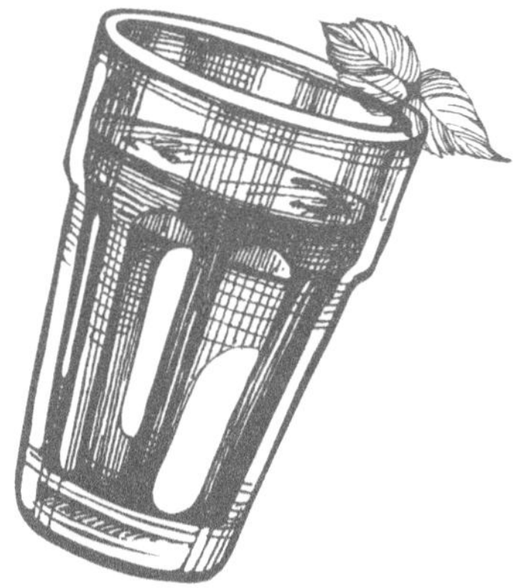

© Copyright 2019 by Michael Vitaloni

All rights reserved.

COPYRIGHT

This document is geared towards providing exact and reliable information with regards to the topic and issue covered. The publication is sold with the idea that the publisher is not required to render accounting, officially permitted, or otherwise, qualified services. If advice is necessary, legal or professional, a practiced individual in the profession should be ordered.

From a Declaration of Principles which was accepted and approved equally by a Committee of the American Bar Association and a Committee of Publishers and Associations.

In no way is it legal to reproduce, duplicate, or transmit any part of this document in either electronic means or in printed format. Recording of this publication is strictly prohibited and any storage of this document is not allowed unless with written permission from the publisher. All rights reserved.

The information provided herein is stated to be truthful and consistent, in that any liability, in terms of inattention or otherwise, by any usage or abuse of any policies, processes, or directions contained within is the solitary and utter responsibility of the recipient reader. Under no circumstances will any legal responsibility or blame be held against the publisher for any reparation, damages, or monetary loss due to the information herein, either directly or indirectly.

Respective authors own all copyrights not held by the publisher.

The information herein is offered for informational purposes solely, and is universal as so. The presentation of the information is without contract or any type of guarantee assurance.

The trademarks that are used are without any consent, and the publication of the trademark is without permission or backing by the trademark owner. All trademarks and brands within this book are for clarifying purposes only and are the owned by the owners themselves, not affiliated with this document

TABLE OF CONTENTS

INTRODUCTION

Green smoothie

Many people think it's difficult to eat many servings of fruits and veggies every day.

Eating salads on a daily basis or bunches of lettuce and spinach may be enough to deter people from pursuing a healthier diet.

Thankfully, there are a variety of pain-free ways to get more green vegetables into your diet without feeling like a bunny rabbit.

Most people who find it difficult to eat green vegetables choose to drink green smoothies instead.

Green are fruit smoothies that have mixed into them leafy greens like spinach or kale.

It may take longer to adjust to the taste, and once you do so, like a green smoothie, you will drink the equal of an entire salad.

Roman lettuce, spinach, kale, carrots, celery, and cucumbers are some common vegetables that can be easily added to smoothies.

Of course, not all of these should be added at once.

To keep it looking fresh, most people who drink green smoothies suggest a ratio of 40 percent to 60 percent fruit.

If you just start drinking green smoothies, pick a mild green like spinach and add a small amount to your smoothie.

Once you have become more used to the taste, you will increase the number of greens you combine.

Green smoothies can also help you eat more vegetables, in addition to increasing your vegetable intake.

A smoothie may include peach, a handful of strawberries, a banana, a few blueberries, and an apple. For one tasty cocktail, this adds up to at least three or four portions of fruit.

Many people thin their smoothies from 100% fruit juice, although some people choose to use water or milk for drinking their smoothies.

Some people thin their smoothies from 100% fruit juice, even though some people want to use water or milk for drinking their smoothies.

Consuming them is also a good opportunity to make your diet healthier, as well as consuming more vegetables and fruit.

It is easy to add healthy fats to it without changing the texture and taste of the drink.

Adding an avocado's meat to a green smoothie will boost the high protein content significantly without harming the taste.

If avocados are difficult to find in your area, consider putting ground flax seeds to your smoothie. Buying whole flax seeds and grinding them at a time is the easiest way to do this.

Only a little teaspoon of coconut oil added to a smoothie will improve the nutritional oomph of the drink significantly.

Most people wonder whether it is easier or worse to drink green smoothies than to juice fruits and vegetables. I still have some significant advantages, although the jury is out.

You're missing the fruit and veggie fibre that's exactly what makes you drink so well.

They make eating all that food convenient for you.

Green smoothies are a concept for meals that many people are becoming increasingly familiar with today.

What was once the average person's unusual or unheard of green drink, popular only to the raw-vegan?

Community, is now becoming a more noticeable staple in many Western homes. For many reasons, green smoothies are gaining popularity, most of which revolve around their awesome nutritional and hence health properties.

But also because of their excellent convenience and taste. We are most often used as a breakfast meal in this way.

Green smoothies, in fact, are my favourite way to start the day and have become the chosen breakfast meal.

Blenders come in many sizes and shapes, and like most kitchen appliances, you get what you pay for. The only way a blender can do you wrong is if the blade easily jams or if the machine is difficult to clean. Shop around and check user reviews when shopping for a product, and be wary of models that fall short in these areas.

All recipes of this book were made using a Vitamix RD Standard blender. This blender is known for its ability to blend everything from frozen fruits to nuts to dry grains. It's certainly worth the high price tag because it lives up to the hype. That said, a pricey blender isn't required to enjoy the recipes in this book.

If you have concerns about your blender's ability to purée with ease, cut harder (or denser) ingredients like nuts, raw beets, carrots, and apples into smaller pieces before adding them to the blender. Also, be sure to add the liquid ingredients first because this always makes for easier blending.

You may be wondering why so many people drink smoothies on a regular basis. They've become a bit of a buzz, suitable for everyone from babies to grannies. Smoothies are the way to optimal health and can be a cornerstone for an overall diet and nutrition makeover. After reading the following list, you'll know why making a habit of drinking healthy smoothies on a daily basis is an outstanding investment in your health.

1. Improve your morning routine. Smoothies are one of the fastest meals on the planet, especially if you invest a little bit of time in properly prepping your ingredients. By just tossing your ingredients in a blender and waiting for the blades to do their magic, you'll have a nutritious, sumptuous meal-in-a-glass at the ready any time of day. Smoothies make particularly good breakfast options for those who are always rushing out the door without having had a solid meal.

2. Break up with the drive-thru. Business lunches, soccer practice, PTA meetings—food is everywhere, and much of it is out of your control. It's easy to let one bad decision lead to others, and before you know it, your car is going through the drive-thru window on the way home from a long day. Having a smoothie each day means that you are in control of at least one of your meals. Why not make it a family affair and ensure that everyone has at least one balanced meal? Drinking a filling smoothie can remove the temptation of indulging in empty calories, and you won't have to go searching for other foods to fulfill your nutritional requirements.

3. Disguise the spinach. While it may not taste like candy, spinach is a green smoothie secret ingredient, and giving it a try will take your nutrition to the next level. Spinach is very low in calories and high in antioxidants, vitamins, minerals, and f iber. It has a mild flavor and can easily be dominated by strongly flavored fruits and additives like nut butters. Smoothies make a great vehicle for hiding other ingredients too like flaxseed, beets, green soybeans, and even broccoli.

4. Add versatility. The best things about smoothies is that you can tailor them to your unique nutritional needs. Healthy smoothies are dense in nutrients and contain a good mix of protein, carbohydrates, and healthy fats. You can modify the types and amounts of ingredients and the calorie count to create a pre- or post-workout smoothie or a smoothie customized to meet your nutritional requirements for breakfast, lunch, dinner, or as a snack. No two smoothies are exactly the same!

5. Vegetables and sneak fruits and into your kids' diets. If your kids' favorite vegetables are French fries and ketchup, you know all too well the challenge of incorporating healthier foods. Blending fruit with milk, yogurt, and nut butters can suddenly turn foods your kids won't eat into something yummy! Kid-friendly smoothies can be made in five minutes or less and are a great way to ensure your kids are getting the nutrients their growing bodies need. Get the kids involved by letting them choose ingredients they like and help with the process of making the smoothies. Pour your kid-friendly smoothies into a thermos for those mornings when you're rushing out the door, or make smoothie pops by pouring them into popsicle molds and putting them in the freezer.

6. Save money. Homemade smoothies are cheap. Buying a healthy breakfast or lunch can cost you close to $10, and buying smoothie at a juice bar can set you back as much as 6 $ a glass. Once you stock your pantry, making a smoothie at home by combining fruits and vegetables will cost you half as much or even less. Frozen fruits and vegetables are some of the most economical options available, and they are just as nutritious as fresh produce—plus, you don't have to worry about them spoiling. So load up your grocery bag with nutritious smoothie ingredients and save yourself some money.

7. Develop an easy, daily habit. Replacing a meal each day with smoothie is an easy habit to develop—much simpler than that marathon you keep meaning to train for and run. Developing a new habit takes practice, the right cues, and the tools you need to be successful. By having your ingredients prepped and cues like a post-it note on your bathroom mirror, you can gradually build a new healthy habit. The fact that smoothies are delicious will make it much more likely that you'll be successful.

8. Have some fun! With the right blender and some basic know-how, you may f ind that making smoothies brings out your creative side. Mixing and matching various ingredients may have you feeling like a modern-day alchemist, noting characteristics, flavors, and textures. Before you know it, you may be posting original recipes online. Loads of people love making smoothies, so why not join the fun?

9. Learn a lot about nutrition. Good fats, bad fats, fiber, protein, vitamins, minerals, antioxidants, probiotics—by learning what constitutes a healthy smoothie, you'll educate yourself on how to follow a healthy diet. By taking note of serving sizes, you'll see how your diet compares to recommendations and what changes you may want to make. You'll also feel the difference in your energy levels and digestion between a diet high in processed foods and one where whole fresh foods take center stage. Then when the blender isn't around, you'll feel more confident in your food choices.

10. Simplify your food decisions. When you make a nutritious smoothie every day, you'll simplify your food decisions. You may also find that you think about food less. Because food is literally everywhere in our society, we're faced with hundreds of food decisions each day. A typical grocery store has upward of 30,000 different items! If you start your day off with a healthy smoothie containing good fats, adequate protein, complex carbohydrates, and enough calories, your cravings will decrease dramatically, simplifying your food decisions.

Smoothies are a best way to get in a few servings of fruits, vegetables, healthy omega-3 fats, fiber, and most importantly, phytochemicals. So aside from being a delicious meal, what health benefits can a well-made smoothie offer?

The following list highlights a few of the more noteworthy ways in which smoothies can improve your health and well-being.

Boost beautiful and healthy hair, skin, and nails. By loading up your smoothie with nutrient-dense ingredients, you will be supplying your body with the raw materials it needs to grow healthier hair and keep your skin and nails healthy. Biotin is a water-soluble B vitamin that is known for its role in promoting healthy hair growth and protecting against dryness. Smoothie ingredients where biotin can be found include bananas, berries, peanut butter, sunflower seeds, oatmeal, avocados, almonds, and Swiss chard. Other essential skin, hair, and nail nutrients include folic acid, vitamin C, lutein, vitamin D, omega-3 fats, and essential amino acids.

Good sources include nondairy milks and yogurts, leafy greens, nuts (especially walnuts) and seeds, and most fruits and vegetables.

Rival the quality and cost of multivitamins. Vitamin and mineral supplements are not regulated by the Food and Drug Administration, nor are they tested for safety before they are put on the market. Supplements can contain much more or much less of the ingredients listed on the supplements fact panel, and there is no way for you to know. Save yourself some money, and use your supplement cash for buying organic fresh and frozen fruits and vegetables to use in your smoothies.

Enhance sleep. Tart cherries are the only natural food sources of melatonin, that controls the body's internal clock to regulate sleep. Research published in the JMF

(Journal of Medicinal Food) has found that tart cherry juice has a modest, beneficial effect on sleep in adults with insomnia.

Bananas, a good source of the natural muscle relaxants potassium and magnesium, are another sleep promoter. Bananas also contain the amino acid L-tryptophan, which gets converted to serotonin, a relaxing neurotransmitter, and to melatonin. Oats, a complex carbohydrate, can ease you into sleep by promoting the release of serotonin and tryptophan, making them a good addition to an evening smoothie. Using chamomile tea as the liquid in your smoothie can also promote a restful night's sleep.

Detoxify your body. You can help your body's natural detoxifying abilities by creating smoothies that contain naturally cleansing ingredients. Doing so will promote the release of water, increase circulation, and keep your kidneys and liver healthy. In addition to including purified water as your liquid, there are a number of delicious ingredients you can use in your daily smoothie to aid your body's natural processes. Detoxifying smoothie ingredients include lemons, limes, watermelons, cranberries, celery, cucumbers, dandelion greens, kale, apples, avocados, beets, pineapples, cilantro, fennel, ginger, and parsley, to name a few.

Fight diseases. A recent study published in the American Journal of Epidemiology investigated the relationship between fruit and vegetable consumption and mortality in 451,151 participants from 10 countries. The results showed that consumption of fruits and vegetables was inversely associated with all-cause mortality. In other words, eat your fruits and veggies to live longer and reduce your chances of developing chronic diseases.

Lose weight more easily. If you are trying to lose weight, then blending up a nutrient-dense smoothie will be your secret weapon. The reason smoothies are such great weight loss tools is because you are in control of the ingredients and the calorie content. It's easy to learn how to assemble a low-calorie, nutritionally balanced smoothie that will keep you full for hours. You can also include add-ins that can increase your metabolic rate and balance your blood sugar. Green tea has compounds that can stimulate metabolism, avocados can increase satiety, chia seeds are full of fiber, and cinnamon can help balance blood sugar levels. If you are the daring type, adding a dash of cayenne, which contains the compound capsaicin, can help curb your appetite.

Recover from exercise. One of the great things about smoothies is that you can tailor the ingredients to your individual nutrient needs and to specific meals or snacks. Instead of buying an expensive powdered protein drink for a postworkout meal, blend up one of the recipes in this book. Contrary to popular belief, you don't need gobs of protein to build muscle. Instead, you need healthy carbohydrates, moderate protein, and healthy fats to replace muscle fuel and to repair and build tissue.

Get your daily allowance of vegetables and fruits. Meeting the recommended intake for fruits and vegetables can be a challenge. By blending two or more servings of each into your daily smoothie, you can ensure that you are on your way to meeting your nutritional goals.

Hydrate yourself. Did you know that high-water fruits and vegetables like celery and watermelon count toward your daily water requirements? Water constitutes about 65% of an adult's body weight, and adequate water is essential for carrying nutrients and wastes throughout the body, maintaining blood volume, regulating body temperature, and keeping our body processes running smoothly. By drinking one healthy smoothie each day, you'll hydrate your body and contribute to your daily fluid requirements.

Improve digestion. Smoothie ingredients are unprocessed, and the fruit and vegetable contents are full of fiber, vitamins, minerals, and antioxidants, which are readily absorbed by your body. Regular consumption of fiber is essential to one's health, and most people don't get enough in their diets, which can result in poor digestion and constipation. Just one healthy smoothie a day can help you meet at least half of the daily recommended intake of 20 to 30 grams of dietary fiber and keep your digestive system running efficiently.

Support your immune system. Fruits, vegetables, and nuts are full of phytochemicals, antioxidants, vitamins, minerals, and healthy fats, all of which are needed to keep your immune system strong. Nutrients that are of particular importance for immunity include vitamins A, B2 , B6 , C, D, and E and the minerals selenium and zinc. Ingredients that you can add to your smoothie for more immune support include probiotics, in the form of cultured soy, coconut yogurt, or kefir; blueberries; cherries; Goji berries; pumpkin; nuts and seeds; and green tea.

Lessen cravings for junk food. When you start the day off with a nutrient-dense smoothie that contains enough calories and some healthy fats, you will find that your cravings for unhealthy fatty foods, especially in the evening, will decrease dramatically. Trying to limit calories or eliminate fat entirely from your diet will just backfire. Doing so may trigger overeating or, even worse, bingeing.

Extend energy and balance blood sugar. With the right mix of ingredients, smoothies can regulate your appetite and keep your blood sugar steady so you don't experience highs and lows during the day. Meals that contain protein, healthy fats, complex carbohydrates, and no refined sugars provide steady fuel to your brain and working muscles, keep your blood sugar balanced, and keep your mood even. Eliminating carbohydrates or fat or restricting calories can lead to low energy, mood swings, fatigue, and low blood sugar. The recipes in this book are all nutritionally balanced and will give you energy to fuel your busy day.

Reach your personal health goals. Whether you are trying to lose weight; increase your intake of fruits and vegetables, healthy fats, or fiber; or decrease your intake of sodium, cholesterol, saturated fats, and refined sugars, smoothies can be tailored to meet your individual health goals. Packed with phytochemicals and nutrients, a smoothie a day can kick the quality of your diet up a notch or two.

ARE YOUR GREEN SMOOTHIES MAKING YOU FAT?

It's no wonder. It's smoothies; it's all rage. Since the early 90s, when smoothie shops began to become as omnipresent as coffee shops.

We became fascinated with their taste, comfort, and wellness halo.

What's better than that? A fast and easy choice to boot for breakfast, lunch, and dinner?

It goes without saying that the smoothie trend started, and soon even fast-food chains added smoothies to their menus.

More recently, it has taken hold of a stronger emphasis on the green smoothie— adding bunches of kale and spinach to your smoothie.

This raises the nutritional content and makes us feel better concerning the food we consume daily in our bodies.

But the story isn't all that's there. It is thought that green smoothies are healthier than their colourful, fruit-laden counterparts, but is that true?

Would your green smoothie be nutrition-free, add to your weight gain, and be responsible for your energy-level dip?

Equality is not produced for all green smoothie recipes. Green smoothies won't automatically make you fat, but the products you add to your green smoothies will add to your diet unhealthy carbohydrates, empty calories, and unnecessary additives.

The impact? A fall in your metabolism that makes it more difficult to drop excessive pounds and lose weight.

5 Widely known green smoothie errors that hamper your weight loss.

We know that mixing a handful of kale is not the most nutritious thing in the world, so many people are adding canned fruit juice, flavoured yogurts.

And even sugar packs to their green smoothie blends to make them tastier and easier to digest. But read our useful tips and most widely known smoothie-making mistakes before you hit the sugar.

Your green smoothies are going to be as delicious, we promise!

1. Use needless sweeteners that are harmful.

Adding a tablespoon of honey will add more than 60 calories to your smoothie.

Which is particularly worrying if you have included a good amount of naturally sweet fruit already.

Weight gain has been correlated with artificial sweeteners, and other foods, such as yogurt and fruit juice.

They contain lots of added sugars that contribute to your drink's glycaemic load.

Alternatively, adhere to a small amount of fruit that helps to sweeten your beverage while adding nutrition. For smoothies, berries are ideal because they are low in sugar but still give natural sweetness.

 You can also choose to substitute the added sugars for a starchy vegetable, such as baked sweet potato or pumpkin puree, without the unwanted side effects.

2. Mixing in dairy products and other products.
Most smoothies made commercially contain some type of milk, such as milk, yogurt, or ice cream.

 In addition to the obvious addition of toxic sugar and processed chemicals, milk products often contain hormones and antibiotics that may cause reactions in those with weakened inflammatory systems.

However, unknowingly, many people have milk allergies or intolerances that can cause headaches or disturb the stomach. Our tip?

 Completely avoid it and instead choose an alternative to milk such as almond milk, coconut milk, or hemp milk.

Looking for thickness to be added? Try to add 1 teaspoon of chia seeds in your next smoothie, this is a natural thickener that helps keep you feeling full.

3. Too much fruit is added to your smoothie green recipe.

To any good smoothie, fruit is a great addition— in the right amounts.

People also include banana on top of mango on top of peach on top of pineapple to disguise the taste of bitter greens and more to make their smoothie palatable.

These are highly glycaemic fruits to eat in moderation.

They contain a lot of vital fiber to help balance their sugar content, but add too much, and you're left with a rapidly metabolized smoothie that left you hungry after a sugar-induced energy crash in an hour.

Instead, choose low glycaemic fruits, such as berries and citrus fruits, and minimize the amounts!

4. Not including the proper balance of complex carbs, fibre, protein, and healthy fats.

Carbs supply fast energy, healthy fats help minimize the risk of chronic disease, protein adds value to the development and rebuild of lean muscle mass in the body.

And also fibre keeps you filled and satisfied— all significant steps in reaching and maintaining a healthy weight.

If your smoothie contains only leafy greens, the advantages of energizing complex carbs and muscle-building protein are missing

If it contains only fruit, the benefits of healthy fats and richer fiber sources are missing.

5. Do not pay attention to the lists of ingredients.

We always recommend that you make your green smoothie at home, so you know exactly what you put in your body.

Yet we agree that life gets in the way sometimes and it's just easier to pick one from your nearest juicer or restaurant.
In such situations, always pay close attention to lists of ingredients and labels of nutrition, as a "green" smoothie is not always the healthiest option.

Search for a list of ingredients including all identifiable ingredients and remember to count those calories!

Stick to the smoothie with less calories (more if a meal is replaced by the smoothie), less than 20 g sugar, and about 10 g fibre.

It takes knowledge and practice to build a delicious, green weight loss smoothie, but never give up!

When you learn the right combination of whole foods, in no time will you be on the way to a healthy weight loss.

How Much Green Smoothie Would I Drink A Day?

At least one green smoothie a day should be drank, preferably in the morning. The smoothie should be about 28 ounces, but not more than 32 ounces.

 It should also provide at least 300 calories so that one of your meals can be replaced with it.

How much Green Smoothie A Day To Lose Weight Will I Drink?

The number of green smoothies you can drink is 2 meal replacement green smoothies per day every day to lose weight.

Such green smoothies need enough calories to fill you up to your next meal to stop hunger and cravings while still helping you lose weight.

The green smoothies will contain approximately 400 calories per 20 oz., 1 pint or 500 ml volume serving size.

The trick to weight loss is to eat less calories than you are consuming. For weight loss, you can get a green smoothie twice a day.

You can substitute a smoothie for breakfast and lunch and have a healthy whole-food meal.

It's crucial that you don't eat on top of drinking the smoothie if you substitute meals with a green smoothie because you don't want the calories to overdo it.

A green smoothie will replace an entire meal with enough calories.

Furthermore, if you drink a smoothie and then eat a meal, your calorie intake will rise and you will not lose weight.
You could also have a smoothie for breakfast and dinner instead of breakfast and lunch.

What Amount Of Smoothies A Day Are Too Many?

It's too much to cover all your meals with a green smoothie every day of the week.

You can find that to substitute meals, you enjoy drinking green smoothies, and that's great. But you don't want a smoothie to cover all of your meals.

If you're going to have three smoothies a day, whether its detox washing or just not having to cook full meals, you're probably going to have to do it for just over a week.

Green smoothies are delicious and safe, but I'm sure you've heard that too much is not good for you. The same applies to the needs of your food.

Is It Good To Be Drinking Green Smoothies Each Day?
Green smoothies help you get your recommended daily fruit and vegetable servings. We contain whole ingredients, unlike juices.

Drinking green smoothies every day is nice, so you've got complete protein and vitamins.

Dietary fibre is essential for excellent colon health by maintaining the proper functioning of your intestines to improve regularity.

Fibre is also a good constipation fighter.

If you have trouble eating enough throughout the day, you may have a green smoothie to replace a meal, or you may have one as a healthy snack to fill you in between.

Because green smoothies offer you antioxidants, minerals, fibre, and vitamins, you also get sugar.

Drinking a green smoothie every day is nothing wrong, but watching the intake of sugar.

Remember, if you're trying to lose weight, be mindful of your smoothie's calories.

The smoothie should not be more than 150 calories for snacking. For a meal replacement, it can be substantially more, but you don't want too many calories.

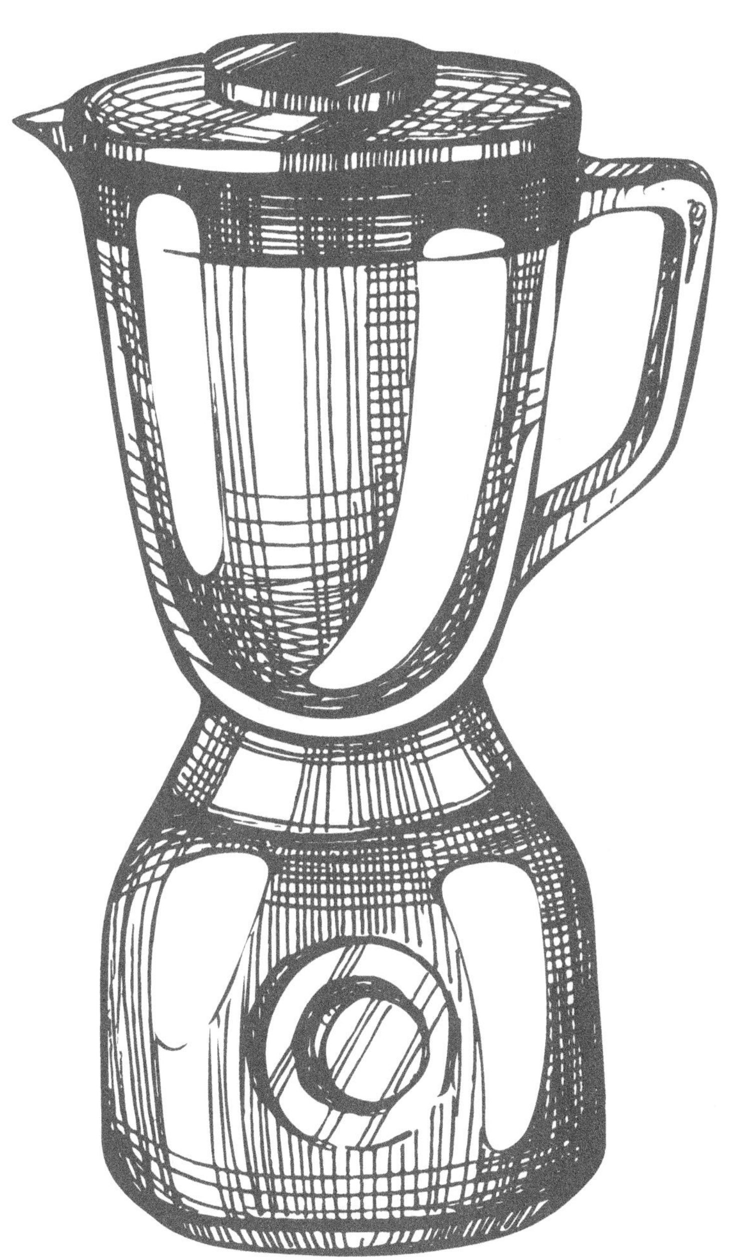

7 DRINKING GREEN SMOOTHIES BENEFIT

1. Hydration

Drinking green smoothies make sure that the water is delivered to you. Every day not everyone is able to drink eight glasses of water.

Nonetheless, you can increase your fluid intake without having to drink plain water if you add more water to your smoothie.

2. Chlorophyll Richness

According to scientists, when you drink green smoothies, you fill yourself with chlorophyll, which has several advantages, such as blood filtering and strengthening the immune system.

Chlorophyll also gives your green smoothie a great energy source to rejuvenate the body.

3. Giving you Radiant Skin

Green smoothies is high in fibre and helps the body get rid of toxins rather than working through your skin.

Vitamin C and E found in green leafy veggies promote healthy skin.

4. Aids in the Focus and Mental Clarity

Antioxidants and carotenoids are present in green leafy vegetables that boost your brainpower and protect your brain as well.

Green smoothies are also full of B vitamins that improve the health and function of your brain and enhance your concentrating capacity.

Always high in folic acid is a green smoothie, which has been proven to help with mental clarity.

5. Encourages weight loss

Naturally And Healthily Green smoothies have low-fat whole foods, vitamins, healthy carbohydrates, minerals and fibres that help you to lose weight quickly and safely.

Green smoothies fill you up so you don't have to eat as much as you can, which is a perfect way to shed pounds.

These are usually low in calories and lower natural sugars than those found in juices and typical fruit smoothies unless they use a green smoothie as a meal replacement.

6. Helps with Total Metabolic Function and Digestion

If you mix veggies and fruits, you break down plant cells that maximize digestibility.

You obtain nutrients by combining vegetables and fruits, which they have a much better delivery to your body than if you were eating a salad.

7. Increases Regular Fruit and Vegetable

Servings it is recommended that you eat at least five to nine regular portions of vegetables and fruits that can avoid cancer and other diseases.

Drinking green smoothies with each glass gives you several servings of fruit and vegetables.

NEGATIVE EFFECTS OF GREEN SMOOTHIE.

Taking too much of it is not good for you, as pointed out earlier. The same is true of green smoothies.

They taste delicious with the fruit that hides the vegetables ' flavour. We are rich in nutrients and have many medical benefits that I have pointed out.

So, How Can Any Adverse Effects Occur?
Okay, because of the absence of chewing, which according to reports, is bad for your overall quality of life, you don't want to drink all your meals daily.

Green leafy vegetables also contain an organic acid called oxalate.

Which, however, binds to certain minerals, is natural in plants and has not been shown to be of any interest to us.

Due to the high oxalate content in them, you should not avoid nutrient-dense foods such as green smoothies.

For a majority of people, it's not a nutrient of great concern. For as long as you want, you can have a smoothie every day.

They're a great way to lose weight, particularly if you replace a smoothie with two meals a day.

Consuming green smoothies has a lot of health benefits.

You do not want to consume them for three meals a day unless you are detoxified, and even then you don't want to lose weight for more than a week.

Whereas a basic green smoothie recipe can truly help with weight loss, supporting the rest of your dietary needs is not enough.

That's why nutritionists suggest that you include plant-based protein, healthy fats and carbs in your usual smoothie mix.

That's how it turns into a meal replacement snack.

It can supplement a plated meal without nutrient skimping

When you substitute foods that are not "empty calories," or those that do not have significant health benefits, you will lose weight.

You can choose from a range of crop-based foods such as leafy greens, legumes, bananas, berries, grains and seeds not only to add spice and colour to your green smoothies but because they are very strong ingredients for weight loss.

Using protein powder will be very beneficial, but I refrain from using highly processed powder mixes as much as possible since they may include artificial additives, which by drinking green smoothies will defeat the purpose of all-natural nutrient intake.

Natural Green Smoothies ' Beneficial Value.

There are many advantages to green smoothies.

And here's a quick guide to more clearly knowing the many benefits: provide healthy meals–no processed foods.

- Provide nutritious meals–no chemicals that are artificial or synthetic.
- Provide an alkaline meal–work to support the balance of acid and alkaline in the body.
- Provide a raw meal–the advantages of living food.
- Come with live enzymes of your own.
- Chlorophyll-rich–multiple health benefits.
- Properties of washing and detoxification.
- Properties that energize and invigorate.
- Fibber-rich–facilitate optimal absorption and removal.
- High in phytonutrients–many benefits for prevention and healing.
- High in vitamins and minerals that are normal.
- A high density of nutrients.
- Low in calories and/or high in calories and nutrients.
- Make a full choice of meal.
- Provide balanced carbohydrates, protein and fats.

- Provide a simple way to add greens to a meal.
- Can be used for breakfast, lunch, dinner, snacks and dessert.
- Easily organic (based on ingredient choices).
- Simple to plan—just take a couple of minutes.
- Pleasant for the entire family.
- Customization and diversification is simple.
- May meet all personal needs, from athletes to loss of weight.
- Excellent vegan and vegetarian diet meal alternative.
- Great meal solution for allergy and gluten-free needs.
- Can be an economical choice of food.
- Convenient —can be consumed, transported, etc. easily anywhere.
- Offer numerous health benefits—lower cancer risk, osteoporosis, diabetes, heart disease, and so on.
- The optimal form of a meal for disease recovery and prevention.

Other essential nutritional values of green smoothie are;

1. Pure nutrition is provided by green smoothies. The amount of vitamins you are going to get depends on the smoothie's fruits and vegetables you choose.

Some fruits and vegetables, however, are rich in A and C vitamins.

Guava also has a high folate content, while avocados provide a high potassium and magnesium content.

2. Green smoothies are much better than juices from fruits or vegetables.

You get vitamins and minerals when you remove nutrients, but no fibre. Nevertheless, the whole fruit/vegetable is used to make smoothies, so you get all the fibre in your drink.

3. Green smoothies are an excellent method to consume your vegetables quickly.

Even though most individuals like fruit, many have difficulties getting their regular veggie needs.

If you make a green smoothie, the flavour of the vegetables is obscured by the fruit taste, so you wouldn't even know the vegetables are there.

4. Green smoothies can be made easily and quickly. The equipment you need is a blender (and a pitcher if you make large quantities and have to put some in the refrigerator).

5. There are inexpensive homemade green smoothies. Buying a juice bar smoothies will set you back a few bucks.

At home, it won't cost you more than a few cents to combine fruit and vegetables.

Every day, drinking glass will give you all the vitamins you need, a much cheaper (and more natural) alternative than buying multivitamins.

6. Green smoothies can be a very good way to "eat" your vegetables to children. You may need to start with a higher proportion of fruit vs vegetables before they get used to the taste.

7. Green smoothies will provide you with a permanent energy source.

Fruits are a good energy source, but consumed alone will only provide short energy bursts (they contain tons of sugars that are easily metabolized).

Green smoothies have low sugar content due to their high veggie content.

8. Green smoothies are very filling but low in calories.

Because they're rich in water and vitamins, they're going to make you feel like you're just having a full meal.

When you try to lose weight, green smoothies can help fight hunger and cravings while making it easier to melt the pounds.

9. it's easy to digest green smoothies.

Because they are already blended and liquefied, the digestion of smoothies is easier.

After all, to absorb the nutrients, the body no longer needs to work so hard to "break down" the food.

People who suffer from indigestion after consuming a heavy meal, as smoothies are filling but sweet, will also benefit.

10. That's right. Green smoothies will hydrate you.

While at least eight glasses of water should be drinking a day, experts believe that most people don't even drink half that amount.

One of the major situations for this is that many people just don't like simple water taste. Just add more water to the mix as you make your smoothie if that suits you.

Without even knowing it, you will be drinking more liquids.

But is that going to taste good?
If you're like others, the nutrition and health benefits might sell you quickly, but you'll have a lot of doubts about the taste.

After all, leafy greens are not normally associated with tasty or mouth-watering meals.

Okay, most people are in for a treat when it comes to the green smoothie.

To begin with, we need to understand that the taste buds of everyone are different. While some people love the banana taste, others dislike it.

So the first trick to making an excellent green smoothie is to tailor it to your taste buds.

The second important feature of taste buds is that the taste buds of most people are filled with the high-intensity sugars, salt and artificial flavours commonly found in most foods today.

Our taste buds change as we turn from a mostly processed food to a mostly natural diet. Once again, they continue to taste food properly, beginning to enjoy natural food, being elevated to true tastes and not filled with artificial foods.

Factors like these make a big difference in how the green smoothie is viewed.

But aside from all these things, as long as you normally get the basic formula to make them, they still taste nice and can easily be called delicious.

Other Essential Nutritional Values of Green Smoothie

Sharper Clarity and Focus

Combining high-fibre leafy greens with fruit provides smooth, stable and consistent energy.

Say adios to the fog of the brain and greet fast wit and focus!

Strengthened Immune System

Mixing high-vitamin A and C fruits and veggies boosts the immune system, the natural defence system for your body against infections and viruses.

Leafy greens support the lymph system, flush out toxins, and decrease inflammation.

Movements Regular Bowel!

The fibre contained in green smoothies acts as an indoor broom to help "move along" digested food inside your body.

We're all on regular day trips to the bathroom and less digestive discomfort.

Regular movements of the intestine can help with bloating, acne, and weight loss over time.

Weight Loss

Green smoothies are filled with vitamins and minerals and packed with fibre, all of which help to reduce weight.

Besides, fibre and good fats keep you full and energized, making it even more convenient to work out.

Green smoothie raw stars frequently lose weight without even attempting to do so.

50 DAYS DETOX/WEIGHT LOSS PLAN

For that graduation party, big wedding, or meeting with your husband, you want to change your body in just 50 days.

Expect substantial weight loss, strengthening muscle tone and increased strength in these seven weeks with sufficient diet and exercise.

Within 50 days, you may not reach your final goal, but you can make great improvement and use it to jump-start lifelong outcomes.

Look to maintain a deficit of 500 to 1,000 calories per day to lose 1 to 2 pounds per week for the most achievable and sustainable outcomes.

 In the first few weeks of the program, you will lose a few extra pounds as your body adjusts, but expect to lose about 14 pounds in the 50 days at most.

Combine exercise and make wise food choices to build the deficit.

How many calories you need daily over the 50 days to lose weight depends on how many calories you need to keep your weight.

 Your calorie needs depend on your age, height, and sex.

Use an online calculator to help you more accurately identify your own.

A diet of between 1,200 and 1,800 calories is considered low-calorie and efficient for women and men weight loss, respectively.

But do not go below these calorie levels or slow down the metabolism.

Dietary weight-loss strategies.
Dietary strategies make it easy for you to lose weight.

Avoid foods with excess sugar, refined carbohydrates and saturated fat to keep up with your low-calorie target.

Calorie-based ditch beverages, such as soda, fruit punch and energy drinks, are mostly sugar and do not contribute to nutrition.

Throughout the week, feel free to mix and match smoothies, and prepare a tasty, healthy and satisfying dinner meal.

Some recipes allow more than one serving, so you can share with others the green goodness, or plan meals ahead with the leftovers.

What Your Meals Look Like.
1. Clean Green Drinks: replace the first week's breakfast and lunch with 2 to 3 clean green drinks.

During the mid-afternoon lull, an energy-boosting juice or green tea can also be drunk.

Drink 10 cups of water every day. And if you need a snack for a pick-me-up?

Choose an apple, a banana, or a few fresh almonds.

Next week is about keeping your health off the table, so be careful!

2. Clean Green Eats: a nice dinner to enjoy. See the options in the following seven-day meal plan.

Continue eating this way for another week if you feel great after this week of clean green drinks and clean food! Gain more strength and lower the pounds.

3. Exercise: Choose a routine that you enjoy. Note that you have to work out every day for at least 30 minutes!

You will find an activity that you love and become addicted to this way of life.

Keeping in shape workout techniques.
A combination of cardiovascular exercise and training in resistance will help you get into shape in 50 days.

Cardiovascular exercise moves large groups of muscles to increase heart rate, break a sweat, and burn calories.

Training in resistance means using free weights, drills, tubing, bodyweight or kettle bells to strain the muscles and make them stronger and more toned.

It also maximizes your metabolism to help you lose pounds by having a higher proportion of muscle mass relative to fat mass.

Use the 50 days in addition to regular exercise to increase the physical activity level throughout the day.

The small non-exercise activity also improves the loss of calories and wellbeing.

Too much sitting, even if you follow the guidelines for physical activity, increases your risk of metabolic disorders and premature death.

If you've got a desk job, get up and walk for five to ten minutes every hour,

Choose the stairs rather than the elevator, fidget, park in the lot further and take on housework as a chance to help you lose pounds.

It includes mixing brief, all-out effort bursts with low-intensity work bouts.

For example, you could do 12 cycles of a sprinting minute on the treadmill, followed by a walking minute.

Do such interval training at two or four workouts a week, but on the other days hold some steady-state exercise to encourage calorie burning.

Too much preparation at intervals wears you out and has rising returns.

Keeping in Shape Strength Training.
Strength training helps to compensate for the normal loss of muscle mass as you age.

This muscle mass loss causes you to feel out of shape and can result in fat gain as a result of slowing down your metabolism.

Do bodyweight exercises for just one set of eight to twelve repetitions when you first start.

Examples of such exercises are squats, lunges, pushes, pull-ups, triceps dips, and crunches. Apply weight, extra workout and more sets after a week or two.

Using weight that feels heavy in your eight-to-12 set at the last repetition and increasing weight as 12 repetitions become fast.

Once you begin strength training for the first time, expect significant muscle tone and strength changes.

This may decrease as you close in on your 50-day mark, but this is normal as improvements become less evident as you become stronger and healthier.

Adjust the routine by increasing weight, rearranging the movements or adding new moves entirely, at least once during the 50 days.

Deadlifts, step-ups, chest presses, and crunches for bicycles and squats for single legs are more difficult movements to put in.

Such changes will help keep you from hitting a plateau that will fully stop your development.

Also offer yourself for specific muscle groups at least 48 hours between workouts to allow repair and recovery, which encourages growth.

Step One: Through portions of your food.
You can begin by eating from small plates, bowls and cups instead of huge 8-and9-inch dinner plates, and don't go back for seconds.

If you're consuming the same meal, the calorie intake will be cut immediately.

Not only will you consume less, but the portions of your food will be automatically changed to be closer to the acceptable serving sizes.

A fruit juice serving is about a half-cup, smaller than a tall tumbler to a 4-ounce juice bottle.

Another tip: instead of coloured and painted dishware, use plain white or cream dishes, as research shows that bright colours inspire you to eat more.

Keep a three-day food diary, complete with what you eat and how much.

Step Two: Do what you love doing.
Would you enjoy dancing? Join for a lesson of salsa. Do you enjoy a good golf or tennis game?

Leave behind and hoof the cart for the caddy and golf.

Love tennis? To get more of a workout, play single tennis instead of doubles.

These activities will make your muscles stronger and calorie burning kick-start.

Many people enjoy walking — and, especially if done regularly, it's a great form of exercise.

 If you're a walker, push yourself to make your walks more intense and longer.

Instead of your usual 15, aim for 20 minutes.

Alternatively, use the talk method to pick up the pace: constantly speak for 30 seconds while you walk, so you breathe more deeply, but don't gasp for air.

Step Three: Go to Burn
To burn fat and lose weight, raise your resting metabolic rate, which is the number of calories the body uses to sustain vital functions.

Raise your muscle mass in order to increase your resting metabolic rate.

Muscle is more active in terms of metabolism than fat, which means more calories are consumed at rest. A pound of muscle consumes at least five to seven calories a day.

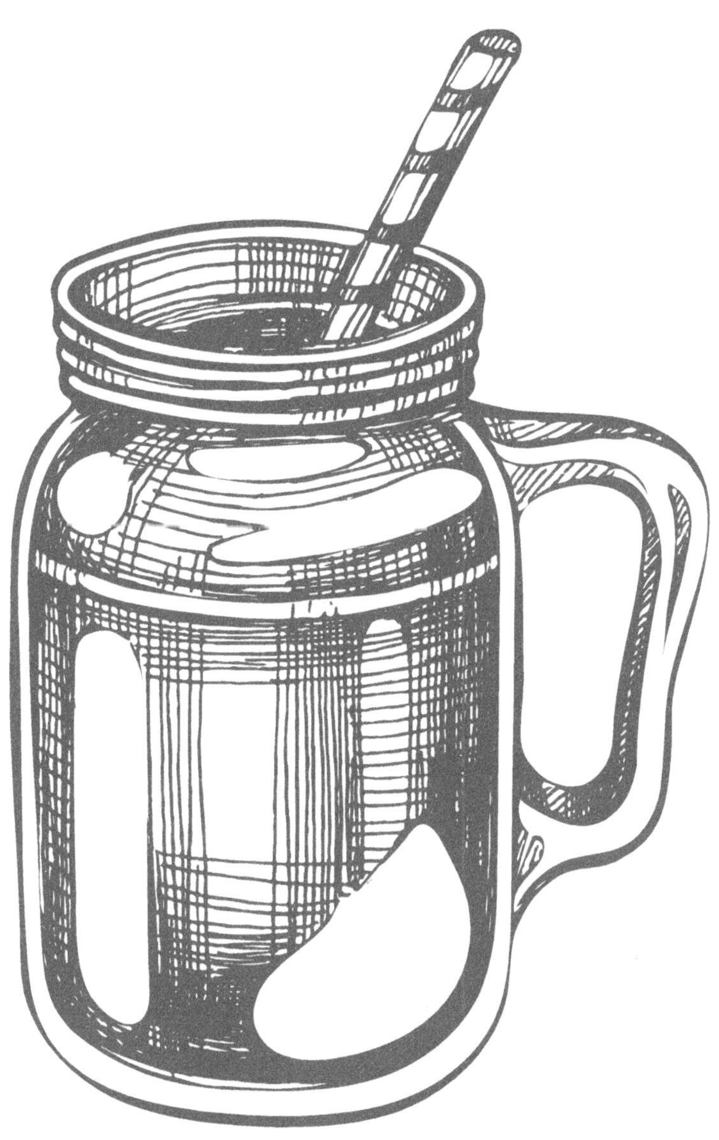

INGREDIENTS

Cherry

Cherries contain both vitamin C and anthocyanin nutrients, a compound linked to inflammatory regulation.

Which means you can help your body heal after a workout by sipping a cherry smoothie.

Blueberries

Wild blueberries have far more fibres and antioxidants than their established relatives, and they are a great source of manganese, a bone-critical mineral.

Often rich in anthocyanin are wild blueberries, which adds a deep blue colour to their nutritional profile.

And while small, wild blueberries deliver big in the taste unit; they actually have a more acute blueberry flavour than the bigger, normal blueberries

Ginger

Why it's good for you: Ginger brings to your smoothie a sweet "zing," while soothing the stomach as well.

Ginger may also help with resistance exercise to decrease inflammation and soreness.

One research found that consuming 2 grams of fresh ginger or ginger spice every day for 11days, 24 hours after the exercise session, reduced muscle pain.

And other work has linked ginger to reduced osteoarthritis pain.

Kiwi

Why it's good for you?

Just one kiwi packs contain reach more than 100 percent of your daily recommended vitamin C value, a crucial antioxidant that helps with the formation of collagen.

Bonus added for this smoothie: mint has a high content of antioxidants.

Almond

Why it's good for you: almonds provide healthy fat, sugar, calcium and nutritional mix.

The bonus healthy ingredients in this recipe include the cacao powder that provides antioxidants.

They also provide powder that delivers protein to help maintain your strength throughout the day.

Carrots

Why they're good for you?

Carrots contribute and make a great ingredient for a smoothie —they're a great source of fibre and vitamin A.

Vitamin A is important not just for healthy skin and eyes, but also for the immune system.

They're a good smoothie add-in for someone who doesn't want their drink too sweet.

Cucumber

Cucumbers are vividly important to add to your diet as they are 95% water and naturally detoxify your body; they are high in vitamins A, B and C; and they contain phytonutrients that have anti-inflammatory, antioxidant and anti-cancer effects.

Thanks to the silica nutrient that helps them grow strong and shiny, they are also a secret weapon for nails and hair.

And they are excellent for soothing irritated or sunburned skin and reviving puffy.

Dark under the eyes because of their cooling and calming effect—simply apply fresh sliced cucumber to soothe the area affected.

Almond Milk Vanilla

Almonds and the milk it produces have many health benefits that people with heart problems, constipation, impotence, diabetes, respiratory disorders, and cough can enjoy.

The nut is full of nutrients. Crush some of the nuts or drink the milk and you will obtain healthy doses of vitamin E, calcium, magnesium, iron and phosphorus.

You'll get a copper, zinc, niacin, and selenium shot as well.

For the skin and anti-ageing, many of these minerals and vitamins are fine.

Vitamin "E" is an effective antioxidant that can benefit youth the skin.

Neutralizing free radical damage is also thought to help keep you healthier at a cellular level.

For your brain, it's good.

In almonds, there are many nutrients that help the human brain.

They are considered an essential food ingredient that is ideal for helping children grow to develop higher levels of intellect.

Regulates the level of cholesterol

Normal almond intake balances the levels of HDL (lipoproteins of high density) and LDL (lipoproteins of low density).

The heart is healthy

The existence in each almond nut of protein, potassium, healthy fats, and magnesium helps to maintain a healthy heart.

The high amount of antioxidants present in almonds helps to reduce homocysteine, allowing fatty plaque to build up in the arteries, thus avoiding heart attacks.

He looks after the fur

It is recommended that almond oil be used with children.

The vitamin E content is believed to support the skin, which is why almond milk is usually found in items of skin beauty such as soap and lotion.

Pumpkin Seed

The greens provide tons of nutrients as well as fibre in this smoothie.

Full facts about nutrients below the recipe add minerals and healthy fats to the pumpkin seeds.

Pumpkin seeds contain a very good source of protein, iron, zinc, manganese, magnesium, phosphorus, copper, and potassium.

Avocado

Avocados, actually known as a fruit, are low in fructose and high in healthy monounsaturated fat (which is quickly consumed for energy).

Research has verified the ability of the avocado to support vascular function and heart health.

Additionally, avocados are very high in potassium (more than twice as much as a banana) and will help balance your essential potassium-to-sodium ratio; contain nearly 20 essential nutrients that promote health, including fibre, vitamin E, B-vitamins, and folic acid.

While consuming them raw, in recipes that call for butter or other oils, you can use avocado as a fat substitute.

Research has also shown that avocados are helpful in controlling blood sugar levels.

May help improve lipid profiles in healthy individuals as well as those with moderate (high cholesterol levels).

Plus, adding an avocado to your smoothie will give you a good chance to absorb more of the antioxidants it contains.

Because of the beneficial raw fat content of avocados, avocado allows the body to consume fat-soluble nutrients more efficiently in other foods consumed together with it.

Kale

Just one cup of kale, along with decent quantities of manganese, zinc, B vitamins, sugar, calcium and potassium, will flood the body with disease-fighting vitamins K, A, and C.

You will also find over 45 separate flavonoids with each serving of kale, which have antioxidant and anti-inflammatory benefits.

Kale is also a good source of sulforaphane and indoles-3-carbinol for the fight against cancer.

Kale has been found to reduce the risk of at least five cancer types, including bladder, breast, colon, ovary, and prostate.

Glucosinolates in kale and cruciferous vegetables break down into products that help protect DNA from damage.

Pineapple

Pineapple contains a bromelain enzyme that improves digestion, reduces inflammation and swelling, and can have anti-cancer effects.

Pineapple, which is rich in antioxidants such as vitamin C, also provides immune support and is an excellent source of manganese, thiamine and riboflavin, which is important for energy production.

Spinach

Spinach is rich in vitamins and minerals, including folate, vitamin A, magnesium, potassium, calcium, zinc and selenium.

Spinach also contains flavonoids that can help protect the body from free radicals, while providing anti-inflammatory benefits and promoting with antioxidant.

Coconut Water

Hawaiians call coconut water "Noelani," meaning "dew from the heavens."

It is a clear, sweet, refreshing liquid (95 percent water) extracted from young, unripe green coconuts.

Coconut water is rich in natural vitamins (B vitamins in particular), minerals, and trace elements (including zinc, selenium, iodine, mercury, and manganese).

For the enzymatic reactions that your cells need to work, vitamins are essential.

Rich of amino acids, fatty acids, proteins and antioxidants.

Rich source of electrolytes and natural salts, potassium and magnesium in particular.

Sweet, low-calorie, low in sugar yet surprisingly sweet contains around one-fifth of the sugar of other fruit juices, such as grape juice or apple juice, as well as some fibre to moderate absorption.

Rich in cytokines or plant hormones that have in humans for anti-ageing, anti-cancer, and anti-thrombolytic effects.

Apple

Apples are a very common type of fruit that contain high levels of dietary fibre, vitamin C, and relatively low-calorie content.

Think of perfect sweet snack, or smoothie ingredient, particularly when on the go.

They are good for weight loss because of their hunger-satisfying nature.

It has been shown that the unique phytonutrient balance found in apples offers strong antioxidant properties. It also have cardiovascular benefits, controlling blood sugar, anti-cancer benefits, helping with asthma.

It also minimizing the occurrence and progression of multi-age diseases.

Your stamina is improved by the antioxidant quercetin, making an apple a perfect snack before you train.

Oats

As various clinical studies have shown, eating oats can help lower cholesterol and protect against cardiovascular disease.

Beta-glucans, a form of fibre in oats, have consistently shown lowering benefits of cholesterol.

Oats are a perfect smoothie ingredient for people with type 2 diabetes with only half a gram of naturally occurring sugar!

Oats add a beautiful green smoothie! We add extra protein, low carb (almost sugar-free) and provide a good source of minerals such as iron, selenium and zinc.

Cashew

Cashew Lime Green Smoothie is a perfect "cleaning" smoothie in the way that is complete with fibre to keep your digestion going.

New cilantro that helps chelate heavy metals in your body, soothe digestion with a touch of fresh mint while ginger gives your metabolism a little heat push and also boosts digestion.

Basically, a healthy digestive smoothie that tastes great and makes you feel fantastic afterwards.

Lemon

Lemons contain high quantities of citric acid, an ingredient that is especially good for increasing bowel movements.

This helps remove waste quickly-so nothing unpleasant has the opportunity to build up.

The separation of all nutrients in food and the removal of waste rapidly prevents bloating to a minimum.

Lemons often eliminates harmful bacteria present in the liver, meaning that the body can generate the enzymes that it requires to flush out toxins.

Furthermore, by serving as a natural diuretic, they keep the urinary tract healthy.

The more regular removal of toxins reduces the risk of building up bacteria that could lead to infections of the urinary tract and other digestive problems.

Psyllium

You should think of psyllium husk as your bathroom buddy as well as encouraging overall digestive health.

It expands in your body and soaks water in your gut, helping your digestive system to move waste.

And scientifically, psyllium allows you to detoxify.

Because... it's not just what we eat, but what we excrete is important to our overall health and well-being—and that's why you need regular bowel movements.

Another benefit of psyllium husk is that to ease constipation, it can be used as a one-off.

Turmeric

In Ayurvedic medicine, turmeric is a major component.

It has been commonly used to treat breathing problems such as cough, runny nose, and sinusitis.

It is also used to treat conditions of the liver, heart, rheumatism, and inflammation.

Turmeric has shown efficacy against various human ailments, including lupus nephritis, cancer, diabetes, irritable bowel syndrome, acne, and fibrosis.

Turmeric can also help protect against cardiovascular disease by potentially reducing cholesterol and triglyceride levels.

Blood sugar levels in diabetic rats have also been shown to decrease.

It has also been shown that I can prevent ulcer formation and defend against Alzheimer's disease.

Brazil nut

Brazil nuts, an important mineral with antioxidant properties, are among the best dietary sources of selenium.

Selenium plays an important role in growth, metabolism, and immune function.

Selenium can improve the antioxidant system of the body in Brazil nuts and prevent oxidative stress.

The liver breaks down selenium into a type of protein called selenoprotein that eliminates excess free radicals effectively.

Free radicals cause oxidative stress, and many chronic health problems, including cancer, have been linked with science.

Tofu

Tofu is not just a good protein source; it also contains all eight essential amino acids.

You will also take some useful minerals such as iron, calcium, manganese, selenium, phosphorus, magnesium, copper, zinc and vitamin B1 by eating tofu.

The level of bad cholesterol is believed to be lowered.

Tofu also produces phytoestrogen with a similar structure to the female hormone oestrogen as a result of which the risk of breast cancer may be reduced.

Green Tea

Green tea is a good source of catechins and antioxidants.

Research has shown that green tea contains three times as many catechins as other standard green tea forms.

Antioxidants can reduce the risk of cancer by preventing and restoring body cell damage and can improve immunity.

<u>**Mango**</u>
Cancer prevention

The fruit pulp of mango contains carotenoids, ascorbic acid, terpenoids, and polyphenols all responsible for the fruit's cancer-preventing effects.

It is also found that mangoes contain unique antioxidants absent from other fruits and vegetables.

Mango's anticancer effects are also due to mangiferin, a compound that is found mainly in the fruit. A study found the suppression of breast cancer by mango polyphenols.

Mangiferin was also found to inhibit the growth of cancer cells of the colon and liver and other tumour cells. For mangoes, the polyphenolic compounds have antioxidant properties.

This also help to reduce oxidative stress (oxidative stress may lead to chronic diseases such as cancer). Moreover, it was also found that these compounds are anti-inflammatory.

Prevent the cancer of the heart

It may help to reduce body fat and control blood sugar by including mangoes in a balanced diet.

 Mangoes have many minerals and phytochemicals that have been shown to have positive effects on body fat and glucose.

Help reduce cholesterol

Mangoes contain pectin which has been shown to decrease levels of serum cholesterol.

Mangiferin (one of the key mango compounds) reduces levels of cholesterol.

Increasing HDL (high-density lipoprotein), the good cholesterol, is also identified.

Can help with diabetes treatment

Mango intake results in lower levels of blood glucose.

This result is due to the presence of a phytochemical, fibre and mangiferin. A mango peel extract has anti-diabetic properties. Mangiferin could have beneficial effects on patients with type 2 diabetes.

Promote Healthy Sex

The fruit is abundant in vitamin E, believed to improve sex drive.Vitamin E and beta-carotene combinations have been shown to enhance men's sperm health.

For male and female fertility, zinc is another essential mineral, and mangoes are rich in it.

Boost Digestion

The presence of fibre that prevents constipation is one of the main reasons mangoes are perfect for digestion. Fibber holds us fresh for a long time as well.

This keeps our colon healthy and facilitates optimum functioning. Furthermore, mangoes contain some digestive enzymes that break down proteins and help digestion.

Fibber was also found to preserve the digestive tract's health, which improves digestion inevitably.

Hemp Seed
Benefit of losing weight

The intake of seeds from the hemp plant works as a natural suppressant of appetite.

Adding these seeds to meals or smoothies, along with side different high-fibre foods, will help cut back excess hunger.

That is due in component to the exceptional of fibre, which encourages satiety and in flip, allows to shed pounds. Lower body weight is associated with fibre consumption. This will be attributed to satiety and the intake of energy after ingesting a high-fibre meal.

Improves the safety of digestion

This seed help to produce enough fibre to maintain your system in a normal way. In fact, this safe roughage combination feeds the gut's probiotics and helps secure a strong immune system.

Their ability to help relieve constipation is one of the benefits of high-fibre foods.

Boosts the protection of hair, skin, and nail

The Health benefit of hemp seed include improvement of dry and dark skin. Including this seeds to your diet plan can to enjoy high advantage of it.

The oil can be used to treat skin ailment such as eczema

Inflammation is raising

Hemp seed helps to reduce inflammation levels naturally and improve the immune system due to its optimal fatty acid profile of omega-3 fats. Hempseed has antioxidant, anti-ageing and immunomodulation effects.

The health of the heart

Hemp seeds help to do all these things. Hemp seeds can boost high blood pressure and cardiovascular health.

Your blood pressure can be drastically reduced by adding two teaspoon of hem seed to a smoothie in the morning.

<u>**Spinach**</u>

Spinach has huge portions of vitamin A.

This moderates the manufacturing of oil inside the pores and skin pores and hair follicles to moisturize the pores and skin and hair. It's far this oil that may be building up to cause zits.

Vitamin A is also important for the increase of all bodily tissues, which include pores and skin and hair.

Spinach and different leafy veggies high in nutrition C are important for the building and preservation of collagen, which presents a structure to skin and hair.

Iron deficiency is a not unusual motive of hair loss, which may be avoided with the aid of a good enough intake of iron-rich foods, consisting of spinach.

Edamame
Edamame is high and low in fat in water.

Protein is the building blocks of life that we all need. It helps repair damaged tissue. The more you can add more protein into your daily diet.

Edamame contains about 17 grams of protein per cup, which is approximately 40% of the recommended daily amount for women.It's amazing! It also supplies around 30% of the daily recommended male quantity and is very low in fat.

For build stronger muscles, Edamame will help

Were you looking for a snack to go with your workout routine? We can't think of anything better than those delicious green soybeans that pack a punch for sure.

Edamame contains 86% more protein than a normal soybean.

A number of gym bunnies and top athletes are beginning to welcome it into their diet for this reason. Every day, a cup of soybeans will help maintain muscle mass, and its calorie content can also flood you with the energy needed to get you through the rigorous workouts.

<u>Pear</u>
Highly nutritious

A medium-sized pear contains nutrients such as calories, protein, carbohydrates, sugar, vitamin C, vitamin K, potassium, and copper.

For cellular function and energy production, folate and niacin are important, whereas vitamin A supports skin health and wound healing.

Pears are also a rich source of important minerals like copper and potassium.

In immunity, cholesterol metabolism and nerve function, copper plays a role, while potassium improves muscle contractions and heart function.

However, these fruits are an excellent source of antioxidant polyphenol that protects against oxidative damage.

As the peel contains up to six times more polyphenols than the flesh, make sure to eat the whole pear.

May promote well-being

By softening and bulking up stool, these fibres help to maintain bowel regularity.

In addition, soluble fibres in your intestine feed the healthy bacteria. As such, prebiotics is considered to be associated with healthy ageing and improved immunity.

Fibre can help relieve constipation, in particular.

Because pear skin contains a large amount of fibre, mixing this fruit unpeeled is best.

Contains beneficial compounds of plants.

Pears offer a lot of beneficial plant compounds that give different shades to these fruits.

For example, some pears are given a ruby-red hue by anthocyanins.

Both compounds can improve the health of the heart and strengthen the vessels of the blood.

There is a reduced risk of heart disease associated with a high intake of anthocyanin-rich foods such as berries.

Green skin pears include lutein and zeaxanthin, two compounds that are needed to keep your vision clear, especially as you age.

Also, the skin is rich in many of these beneficial plant compounds.

Have anti-inflammatory properties.

Your health may be harmed by chronic or long-term inflammation.

Several major reports relate the high intake of flavonoids to a lower risk of heart disease and diabetes.

This effect can be attributed to the anti-inflammatory and antioxidant properties of these compounds.

However, pears are packaging some vitamins and minerals, such as copper and vitamins C and K, which are also battling inflammation.

May have the properties of antioxidants.

In response to stress or injury, their production increases.

Your body will be in a state of oxidative stress when there are too many free radicals, which can kill your cells and increase the risk of disease.

Can help prevent the stones of the kidney.

It is necessary to drink enough fluids to avoid kidney stone. If calcium, oxalate and other compounds are combined to form crystals in your urine, kidney stones form.

Such stones can then be shaped. Many individuals, however, are more likely than others to acquire them.

Can Heart Health Aid Drinking coconut water can be useful in reducing the risk of heart disease?

Blood cholesterol and triglycerides are reduced by people who consume coconut water. They also experience substantial declines in liver fat. Proves muscle contractions and heart function.

However, these fruits are an excellent source of antioxidant polyphenol that protects against oxidative damage.

 As the peel contains up to six times more polyphenols than the flesh, make sure to eat the whole pear.

What else is included

May promote well-being.

By softening and bulking up stool, these fibres help to maintain bowel regularity.

In addition, soluble fibres in your intestine feed the healthy bacteria. As such, prebiotics is considered to be associated with healthy ageing and improved immunity.

Fibre can help relieve constipation, in particular. Because pear skin contains a large amount of fibre, mixing this fruit unpeeled is best.

Contains beneficial compounds of plants.

Pears offer a lot of beneficial plant compounds that give different shades to these fruits.

For example, some pears are given a ruby-red hue by anthocyanins.

Both compounds can improve the health of the heart and strengthen the vessels of the blood.

There is a reduced risk of heart disease associated with a high intake of anthocyanin-rich foods such as berries.

Green skin pears include lutein and zeaxanthin, two compounds that are needed to keep your vision clear, especially as you age.

Also, the skin is rich in many of these beneficial plant compounds.

<u>Dandelion green</u>
Highly Nutritious

Dandelion greens are highly nutritious plants from root to flower, loaded with vitamins, minerals and fibre.

Dandelion greens also provide major minerals, including iron, calcium, magnesium, and potassium.

The dandelion root is rich in carbohydrate inulin, a plant-based source of soluble fibre that promotes the development and maintenance of a healthy bacterial flora in your intestinal tract.

Contains potent antioxidants

Dandelion is filled with strong antioxidants, which can explain why this plant has such large applications for safety.

Antioxidants are compounds that either neutralize the body or prevent free radicals from having negative effects.

There are too many free radicals that lead to disease growth and accelerated aging. Therefore, antioxidants are essential for a healthy body.

Dandelion contains high levels of antioxidant beta-carotene, known to provide heavy cell damage and defines against oxidative stress.

These are also rich in another group of antioxidants called polyphenols, found in the flower at the highest concentration, but also in the roots, leaves and stems.

Can Blood Sugar Help Regulation

Chicoric and chlorogenic acid are two bioactive compounds in dandelion.

These can be found in all parts of the plant and can help reduce blood sugar.

Such compounds will increase the secretion of pancreatic insulin while also improving the absorption of glucose (sugar) in muscle tissue. This process leads to increased insulin sensitivity and lower blood sugar levels.

Lime
Skin Care

Lime juice includes healthy acids and allows put off dead cells whilst carried out to the skin. It builds collagen, rejuvenates the pores and skin, and improves everyday texture.

Eating vitamin C protects the pores and skin from infections in addition to treatments rashes, acne, pimples, bruises, and blemishes, flavonoids contained in limes.

Additionally it inhibit microbial boom, hitch helps save you gum bleeding.

It fights skin harm brought about due to sun, dirt, and pollution.

Its antioxidant and astringent residences can assist lessen wrinkles, in addition, to decrease dark spots, skin tan, and open pores.

You may create a fresh bathing revel in through simply including this juice for your tub.

It also allows the lessening frame scent. For a while, the usage of lime has been a remedy for scurvy, a sickness because of Vitamin nutrients C deficiency.

Its miles characterized thru commonplace infections that display everyday cold signs and symptoms, cracked lips, and lip corners.

Aids in Digestion

Limes have an irresistible aroma, which may also moreover motive your mouth to water. This aids number one digestion (the digestive saliva floods your mouth even in advance than you flavour it). The herbal acidity of lime does the relaxation.

At the same time as they destroy down the macromolecules of the meals. The flavonoids stimulate the digestive tool and increase the secretion of digestive juices, bile, and acids.

This additionally stimulates peristaltic movement which actions the meals at a few degrees inside the gut.

The sufficient quantity of acid found in lime allows easily the excretory gadget. The roughage in lime can also moreover resource in presenting relief from constipation.

An overdose of its juice with salt moreover acts as an exquisite purgative without any element effects, thereby relieving constipation.

Moreover, drinking a tumbler of heat lime water approximately half-hour earlier than meals can assist prevent heartburn or acid reflux disease sickness signs?

Weight reduction

The essential oils located in lime prevent weight benefit and extra meals intake. Additionally, the citric acid found in its miles a first-rate fat burner.

A pitcher of heat water with the juice of an entire lime can be powerful as a first-rate weight reducer.

The way to use: eat two glasses of warm water with lime juice a day to acquire blessings in a few days.

Manages Blood Sugar

The excessive levels of soluble fibre discovered in lime make it effective in helping to regulate the frame's absorption of sugar into the bloodstream.

These permits lessen the prevalence of blood sugar spikes which is probably a critical risk to diabetic sufferers.

Additionally, limes and one-of-a-kind citrus culmination have a low glycaemic index

This means they may not motive any large or surprising spikes in glucose ranges.

Prevents heart illnesses

Food rich in nutrition C has a shielding effect on coronary heart ailment.

Moreover, soluble fibre and limonin located in limes help decrease blood pressure.

This permits reduce the irritation of the blood vessels and similarly aids in decreasing the chance of coronary heart diseases.

Also, potassium and magnesium in limes improves blood flow and boosts coronary heart health.

Food plan C in lime juice and lime peels may additionally help decrease ischemic stroke dangers.

It moreover enables sluggish down the progression of coronary heart ailments like atherosclerosis with the aid of lowering fatty streaks in arteries.

Hesperidin, a flavonoid present in lime, allows lower cholesterol and triglyceride stages within the frame it truly is a few different coronary heart-healthful advantage!

Anticancer capacity

Citrus give up result may additionally comprise precious anti-most cancers residences. Lime juice consumption can be beneficial for maximum cancers treatment.

This is because of its ability to scavenge loose radicals and reduce oxidative stress. Antioxidant-packed phytochemicals like flavonoids, flavones, triterpenoid, and limonoids in lime have robust cancer-preventing houses.

They're able to prevent the growth of diverse cancer cells preventing colon, breast, and prostate, pancreatic, stomach, lungs, kidneys, and blood cancer. It is also able to remove maximum cancers cells in some cases.

Relieves infection

The citrus end result, in popular, has homes and may be used for some of the anti-inflammatory problems.

One of the many reasons for arthritis is an additional construct-up of uric acid in the frame. The citric acid located in limes is a solvent in which uric acid can dissolve. Increasing citric acid in the body permits get rid of extra uric acid from the urine.

Prevents Kidney Stone

The citric acid in glowing or targeted lime juice facilitates take away and save you kidney stones with the aid of manner of growing urinary citrate and urine amount.

Boosts Immunity

Lime strengthens the body's line of protection and enables push back infections and illnesses like malaria, diarrhoea, and pneumonia.

Moreover, vitamin C inside the citrus fruit permits to war coughs and colds and boosts the body's common immunity.

Will Growth Iron Absorption

Food vitamin C in lime whilst paired with food rich in iron, allows maximize the body's capability to take in iron. The ones suffering from iron-deficiency anaemia signs like — dizziness, brittle nails, hair loss, and fatigue want to preserve in mind such as lime to their diet!

Heals Peptic Ulcer

In addition to Vitamin nutrient C, lime includes unique compounds called flavonoids.

Which also have antioxidant, anti-carcinogenic, antibiotic, and detoxifying residences. The acids in lime react with the gastric juices of the stomach ensuing in alkaline reactions.

The flavonoids and the alkaline response together stimulate the recovery technique of peptic and oral ulcers.

Treatment from respiration troubles

The flavonoid-rich oil. This is extracted from limes is substantially used in anti-congestive pills which include balms, vaporizers, and inhalers because of the presence of kaempferol.

Vitamin C also prevents the cause of asthma due to air pollution.

<u>Cilantro</u>

In case you don't normally consume ingredients along with carrots or candy potatoes that comprise excessive quantities of vitamin A, your body may not be getting sufficient.

The hassle is, your body desires nutrition A for a healthy immune machine, eyes, pores and skin, and mucous membranes. You certainly don't want any of these objects performing at a suboptimal level because of a simple deficiency.

That's why it's a top-notch concept to add foods on your eating regimen that comprise nutrients A. Cilantro is the kind of foods.

In reality, just a ¼ cup (sufficient for a garnish) can provide 270 IU of this critical nutrient to assist keep your eyes sharp.

Allows getting rid of harmful Heavy Metals

Although it's not as effective as zeolite for detox, studies propose cilantro can assist rid heavy metals from your body.

That is large seeing that most people are unknowingly uncovered to heavy metals on a normal basis. Over the years, pollution can increase to your tissues where they are able to wreak havoc at the body.

Helps coronary heart health

The good news is that taking smoothies rich in leafy veggies can guard your coronary heart. And cilantro is any such elements which can provide you with a similar area closer to oxidative damage. Evidence suggests that the phytochemicals in cilantro ought to guard your heart against oxidative damage supporting to preserve it healthy.

Balance Blood Sugar Ranges

Cilantro moreover indicates the capability to help stability blood sugar degrees, giving a few different excellent causes to add it to salads and smoothies.

Cilantro can be used to assist and manipulate diabetes, given how destructive advanced levels of glucose inside the frame can be. Anybody can advantage from preserving blood sugar degrees balanced.

It can also help you maintain regular power rangers at a few stages in the day.

Cilantro may additionally ease anxiety

Is an unfortunately not unusual hassle that human beings war with? Cilantro can be a natural manner to locate comfort.

A cilantro extract is certainly as powerful as anti-tension drugs like diazepam for lowering anxiety.

Considering maximum anxiety pills include a hefty list of side outcomes. Cilantro may be an interesting opportunity to remember along with your health practitioner.

Need to prevent meals poisoning

Possibilities are you've skilled food poisoning in the end on your existence.

Notorious nausea, muscle aches, bloodless-sweats, and headaches you get several hours after a questionable meal ought to make you miserable to mention the least.

However, evidence indicates you could lessen your probabilities of having food poisoning by way of using consuming cilantro with a meal, in particular via a smoothie. Cilantro is particularly protective in the direction of listeria—a bacteria that frequently motives what we realise as food poisoning.

Protects your mind

Ailments of the mind together with Alzheimer's or Parkinson's, are believed to be related to subjects: continual irritation and oxidative damage.

Amazingly, proof shows that cilantro can defend your thoughts from every.

First, it consists of many antioxidants along with nutrients and the flavonoid quercetin which might be protective in competition to oxidative stress.

Secondly, diets immoderate in spices together with turmeric, clove, ginger, garlic, and cilantro drastically lessen persistent irritation.

Supports imaginative and prescient with vitamin A.

In case you don't typically devour ingredients which consist of carrots or candy potatoes that comprise immoderate amounts of nutrition A,

Your body may not be getting enough.

The hassle is, your body desires weight loss plan A for a healthful immune gadget, eyes, pores and skin, and mucous membranes. You surely don't want any of this stuff performing at a suboptimal degree due to an easy deficiency.

That's why it's a fantastic idea to add ingredients on your food regimen that comprises nutrition A. Cilantro is the type of meals.

Grapes

Grapes packed with antioxidants

They are an antioxidant powerhouse—they contain a wide variety of phytonutrients from carotenoids to polyphenols.

Such phytonutrients assist in preventing many cancers and helping to preserve the fitness of the pores and skin.

Resveratrol is thought amongst polyphenols for its excellent houses together with inhibiting the formation of unfastened radicals.

Although it can cause cancer and dilate blood vessels to ease blood drift and decrease blood strain.

Remember the fact that in seeds and skin, the antioxidant content is the largest, so make use of it.

Prevents skin troubles

Resveratrol is found to save you signs of ageing and different pores and skin problems.

Whilst paired with a famous benzoyl peroxide zits medicinal drug, resveratrol battles the microorganism-causing acne.

High Potassium supply

The nutritional breakdown of grapes indicates that there may be 191 mg of potassium in step with 100 grams of fruit. Excessive potassium intake and a discount in sodium content material will help the frame in lots of approaches.

Regularly, potassium counteracts sodium excess.

In maximum instances, a low-sodium-excessive-potassium food plan has been proven to be good for excessive blood stress, high cholesterol and heart health.

A bloated belly can cause many issues associated with fitness.

Lowering the consumption of salt and focusing on potassium-rich fibre can also help to get a flat stomach.

<u>Peaches</u>
Cancer Prevention

Packed with vitamin C and phytochemicals, peaches are a sweet maximum cancers fighter.

Vitamin "C" acts as an antioxidant to fight off free radical damage to cells that may cause maximum cancers. And other than their antioxidant houses, peaches have powerful phytochemicals which are probably identified for their most cancers-preventing homes.

This also include reducing inflammation, stopping DNA damage and decreasing oxidative stress.

Diabetes

For folks who be afflicted by diabetes, counting carbs and proscribing blood sugar spikes is kind of a complete-time mission.

However, thankfully, a medium-sized peach only has 14 grams of carbs, which means you may experience it without worrying approximately sending your blood sugar sky excessive.

Other than the moderate amount of carbohydrate awesomeness, peaches actually have a respectable amount of fibre-that is important for controlling blood sugar stages and keeping you complete. (No longer to mention, the fibre will help keep your digestive track running easily!)

Imaginative and prescient

With an exquisite amount of vitamins A, peaches are amazing for keeping healthy eyes. Nutrition A is crucial for eye fitness because it can save you night time imaginative and prescient and aids with healthful mucous membranes. So, we can be taking all the peach pie we are able to get.

Coronary heart health

Thanks to their high potassium content material, peaches must be part of your coronary heart-healthful weight loss plan (in the event that they aren't already).

Research endorses that lowering sodium consumption and growing potassium levels can sell a healthful coronary heart. Not handiest does potassium lessen the outcomes of sodium

But it decreases the tension in blood vessels and decreases blood strain-a threat thing for cardiovascular disorder.

<u>Greek yoghurt</u>
The power of Protein

Protein is important for correct health. It is essential to cellular increase, building muscle, and repairing tissue.

As you age, you need extra protein to hold your pores and skin healthy and to combat off infection.

Greek yoghurt is a wonderful way to reinforce your protein levels at equal time as maintaining off heavy substances like meats. Have it for breakfast and add in a handful of walnuts and blueberries, or in the mixture as a smoothie.

Use it as an opportunity for bitter cream on top of chilli or baked potatoes.

Probiotics keep you normal

Greek yoghurt is full of probiotics. Those are microorganisms which include microorganism and yeast.

These generally live on your intestines, and having microorganisms nicely in your intestines helps maintain you healthy.

Without wholesome stability of the right microorganism from probiotics, an excessive amount of awful bacteria can boom and purpose damage to our immune structures.

Probiotics are for the digestive tool, and specifically beneficial to individuals who be via situations along with side irritable bowel syndrome.

Get Your B12 right here!

Nutrition B12 is essential for energy and healthy mind characteristic, and Greek yoghurt is full of it.

Many pick to supplement diet B12 into their weight-reduction plan, but Greek yoghurt gives an effective, natural possibility. Vegetarians are frequently poor in B12 as it typically is determined in meats.

Greek yoghurt is a terrific, meat-unfastened manner of functioning greater for your diet regime.

Potassium Balances Our Sodium

Maximum people have manner too much sodium in their food regimen.Now not satisfactory is Greek yoghurt low in sodium, it's also excessive in potassium.

What does one should do with the alternative?

There must be right stability amongst sodium and potassium in the frame, and Greek yoghurt assist you in maintaining the right proportions.

Honey

The whole thing has a shelf lifestyle, right? Honey does not, due to its chemical make-up and shape.

Honey has antifungal, antibacterial and acidic qualities that make it hard for the substance to damage.

Prevention of Gastric Ulcers

Stomach ulcers is one of the most important afflictions of the modern-day day bad weight-reduction plan and excessive alcohol intake.

Pylorus is a shape of microorganism. This is accountable for the majority of gastric ulcers.

Another time honey's powerful antibacterial houses act as each a symptomatic remedy and preventative.

Chia seeds
Weight Loss

Meals which can be excessive in fibre assist people to experience complete for longer, and they'll be usually lower in energy.

This seed also contains nearly 5 grams of fibre in line with a tablespoon, and their high degrees of omega-3-fatty acids and alpha-linoleic acid can be useful for weight loss.

The seed also can be fed on as a gel at the same time as mixed with water.

This motives it to digest more slowly in the body, probable preventing starvation for an extended period.

Cardiovascular ailment and cholesterol

Prolonged fibre intake has been verified to decrease blood strain and cholesterol levels.

Even a modest 10-gram consistent with day growth in fibre consumption reduces LDL, or "lousy" cholesterol, further to general cholesterol.

Recent studies have proven that nutritional fibre may moreover play a function in regulating the immune device and infection.

 In this way, it could lower the chance of infection-related situations inclusive of cardiovascular illness, diabetes, maximum cancers, and weight issues.

<u>**Almond butter**</u>
 Almond butter is a superb supply of the healthful fat our bodies want. Those fats are associated with lowering the threat of heart ailment.

Eating almonds gives antioxidant movement from nutrients E and helps lower cholesterol.

A small serving of almond butter consists of a beneficent quantity of magnesium which enhances coronary heart fitness.

By promoting the go together with the waft of blood, oxygen, and vitamins and potassium, important for proper blood stress and heart fitness.

Eating almond butter facilitates blood sugar strong. For example, carboy first rates that could cause blood sugar to increase and crash).

The low-glycaemic index and protective antioxidants of almonds makes almond butter a sensible desire for the ones at hazard from diabetes.

 Due to the fact they don't purpose a sharp increase in blood sugar and insulin whilst fed on.

They even seem to assist whilst you eat them at the side of ingredients that have a better glycaemic index.

Clementine
High Content Material of Nutrition C

Clementine is a supply of weight loss program C which need to be taken externally due to the fact the frame could not produce it.

The day by day consumption of Clementine presents vitamins C to the body with the resource of stopping the chances of several ailments along with side hardening of arteries and excessive blood strain.

Moreover, it allows to promote the immune tool and counteract cardiovascular troubles.

It makes the immune device strong in order that body might be capable of counteracting viruses which might be the cause for deadly diseases and promotes disease-resistant body.

It also assist in launching energy at some point of metabolism technique.

Wheatgrass powder

Wheatgrass assist you to manipulate weight because it works to manipulate the thyroid gland.

The vitamins observed inside wheatgrass additionally help to regulate food cravings and assist save you binge eating. Wheatgrass is a digestive resource way to its enzymes, amino acids, and vitamin B content material.

It's been showed to help with conditions which include heartburn, indigestion, ulcers, and irritable bowel syndrome (IBS). It moreover facilitates to sell wholesome intestinal plant life through boosting the wide variety of pinnacle bacteria that your gut calls for advanced health feature.

Wheatgrass has anti-ageing homes way to its catalase content material together with specific antioxidants.

The chlorophyll decided in wheatgrass permits to provide greater oxygen on your blood which aids your immune tool function.

It also acts as an energy booster.

<u>**Matcha powder**</u>
Sufficient Antioxidants

Matcha powder is loaded with antioxidants called polyphenols, which have been connected to a discounted hazard of maximum cancers and coronary heart disorder.

Further, antioxidants fight off reactive oxygen species within the body that wreak havoc on frame cells. In quick, antioxidants guard and save you cells from oxidative harm.

Immune resource: because of the fitness-boosting antioxidants, amino acids and other compounds contained in matcha. Studies suggest that matcha has an effect at the body and may beautify standard immune responses.

Mood Boosting: studies suggests that the serotonin and the amino acid L-theanine determined in matcha also can assist in lowering tension and improving one's common mood.

Wholesome heart: studies show that the antioxidants determined in matcha may work to disrupt cholesterol absorption from food within the gastrointestinal tract, consequently contributing to lower (horrible cholesterol) ranges circulating via the blood.

Fights irritation

Positive proteins in Romaine lettuce, help manage inflammation.

Vegetables (like lettuce) that are rich in nutrition ok can dramatically decrease inflammation.

You could typically encompass two cups of raw leafy vegetables to your food plan on a regular foundation. Other food plans ok-rich vegetables encompass kale, broccoli, spinach, and cabbage.

And the darker the lettuce, the extra antioxidants it has – which further make contributions to its houses.

Lettuce is one of that pain-secure food. This indicates the veggie in no manner contributes to arthritis or associated painful conditions.

Aids weight loss

One number one reason lettuce can be an excellent weight reduction meals is energy – one serving of lettuce includes simply five energy.

 Moreover, lettuce helps bridge the micronutrient hole. This is otherwise difficult to achieve on a low-calorie eating regimen.

Unbalanced risky food regimen can harm blood vessel and result in haemorrhage and lesions.

Soy milk is densely rich in omega 6 and omega 3 fatty acids in addition to phyto-antioxidants that could fortify the blood vessel lining and preserve free radicals assaults at bay.

The ones compound also enhance the ability and fluidity of your blood vessels.

Broccoli
Preventing most cancers

Cruciferous veggies – specifically broccoli- assist lessen the chance of cancer and slow its development.

That is due to the excessive stage of sulforaphane observed in broccoli.

Helping coronary heart fitness

Coping with your intake of fibre-rich substances lets in lessen and prevent heart illness.

Broccoli, being complete of antioxidants and fibre can assist combat in opposition to the danger of coronary heart attacks and cardiac arrest.

Broccoli moreover helps with the hazard of immoderate cholesterol that is a chief motive of coronary heart failure.

With its excessive degrees of soluble fibre, it's very powerful in supporting to reduce the cholesterol.

Improving Immunity

Another benefit of broccoli is its capacity to reinforce the immune system.

This is the most important device in protecting the body in opposition to viruses, microorganism, and diseases.

One cup of broccoli has a hundred thirty 5% of every day endorsed charge of food plan C.

Broccoli is packed with nutrition C, that's a vital factor in defensive our bodies in opposition to contamination and sickness.

 In choice to just grabbing orange juice to combat that bloodless, bear in mind growing a broccoli smoothie.

<u>Mustard greens</u>
Fitness blessings

Research has proven that growing your consumption of inexperienced leafy vegetables, like mustard greens, can drastically reduce your danger for numerous forms of cardiovascular sickness.

In addition, replacing starchy elements with the one's varieties of greens allow you to manipulate your blood sugar and keep a healthful weight.

Mustard vegetables also are ideal in your frame due to the critical advantages furnished with the aid of the nutrients they comprise.

The mineral in mustard veggies is critical for top health.

 Mustad gren is fat-soluble nutrition that enables with blood clotting capabilities inside the body and is mainly vital for folks that take blood thinners.

Vitamins adequate moreover boosts bone fitness.

A vitamin k deficiency may additionally place you at greater danger for osteoporosis.

Nutrition A is fat-soluble nutrients that let you preserve actual imaginative and prescient, immune function, and healthy pores and skin.

Vitamin A is crucial for proper cell division and differentiation.

<u>**Collard vegetable**</u>
Vitamins Records

Collard veggies include a big amount of calcium, weight-reduction plan a, nutrients C, nutrition ok, manganese and folate.

Even as eaten in a raw kingdom, they help to detoxify the frame and reduce cholesterol.

Collards are complete of antioxidants, which might also have effective anti-growing old and anti-cancer residences.

Additionally, they assist in altering blood sugar and defend the body in opposition to viral infections. Vegetables also are high in chlorophyll, so that you can boom the frame's pH ranges.

Blood Alkalinity

Collard vegetables are alkaline meals. By means of ingesting ingredients that are alkaline, you could enhance your frame's pH diploma, stopping ailment and premature degeneration.

While the body is alkaline, illnesses have a difficult time surviving.

Chlorophyll, which gives collard veggies their deep, wealthy colouration, is what makes them an alkaline food.

Chlorophyll also facilitates body sores to heal fast, eliminates frame odours and improves vision in individuals who devour it regularly.

Enhance Your Immune system

Consuming vegetables can appreciably boom your immune tool.

Inexperienced leafy vegetables, collectively with collard veggies, match a human's required nutrients goals perfectly;

Therefore, while consumed in large quantities, they can dramatically affect your fitness. The manner to boost your immune device is to chorus from cooking the leaves.

Cooking destroys maximum of the dietary residences important for an immune system enhance, so constantly make your smoothies using uncooked collard inexperienced leaves.

Agave nectar

This plant is used for excessive fuel, prone digestion and constipation.

This plant is likewise used to offer alleviation from stomach contamination, ulcers, jaundice, stomach inflammation and liver ailments.

Agave efficaciously promotes perspiration and gives remedy from immoderate fever.

Girls with menstrual problems want to devour agave.

The Agave Syrup

Healthy supply in your body. The number one of herbal agave's advantages, and particularly that of agave inulin, is its 100% dietary fibre content.

This makes it a low-glycemic and rather nutritious sweetener.

Herbal agave nectar vitamins specialists advise it as a sugar substitute for diabetics as it does now not motive a spike in blood sugar that maximum traditional sweeteners are associated with.

Furthermore, the fibre content material complements digestive health because its miles a prebiotic, which helps foster the exceptional bacteria our bodies rely on.

As an end result, the frame absorbs more calcium and magnesium, ultimately enhancing bone health.

Natural Agave Syrup Make Experience for Your Pockets

Every maple syrup and agave are famous and healthier options to sugar.

Which begs the query, why selected Agave, above the two? Aside from several of the nutritional houses, a brought benefit of natural agave syrup is pure economics.

It takes loads of litres of raw maple sap to offer numerous litres of geared up-to-devour, completed maple syrup.

This effects in maple syrup being two instances as agave syrup and a much less economically viable choice for those who plan on substituting it for sugar on an ordinary basis.

<u>**Cayenne pepper**</u>
Relieving pain

Capsaicin, the energetic ingredient observed in cayenne peppers, May additionally have ache-relieving houses.

One evaluation of research into cayenne pepper's capability to reduce pain concluded that it might have advantages as long-time period analgesia.

This can also occur without bringing about different sensory modifications.

Burning strength and suppressing urge for meals

There are numerous products containing cayenne pepper that decorate metabolism and promote weight reduction.

Relieving congestion

Cayenne pepper is frequently used as a home remedy for coughs, colds, and congestion.

There aren't any studies to useful resource this use.

However, cayenne can also additionally help to quickly relieve congestion via shrinking the blood vessels within the nostril and throat.

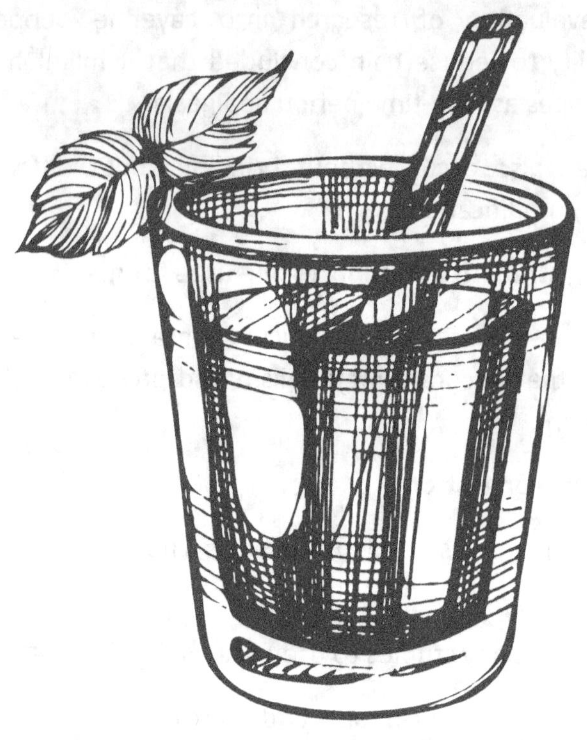

LIST OF RECIPES

Day 1
Green Dreams

HIGH-FIBER and HEART-HEALTHY

Broccoli may seem like an unusual smoothie ingredient, but the bitterness is tempered by the addition of the flavorful berries.

Tip: Avocados are rich in monoun saturated fats and can increase feelings of satiety.

1 cup unsweetened, protein-fortified almond milk

2 tablespoons ground flaxseed

1 Medjool date, pitted ½ cup avocado

1 cup frozen spinach ½ cup frozen broccoli ½ cup frozen blueberries

1 cup ice

In a blender, combine the almond milk, flaxseed, date, and avocado and process into a thick paste.

Add remaining ingredients and blend until smooth. If smoothie is too thick, add liquid and thin to desired consistency. Serve right away.

Nutritional info: calories: 390, fat: 19 grams, carbs: 36 grams, fiber: 18 grams, protein: 12 grams

Day 2
Green Boost

JOINT-SUPPORTING and BEAUTY-BOOSTING

Hydrate and boost your immune system with this green smoothie. Pumpkin seeds are high in immuneboosting zinc and blood-building iron, two minerals that can be tricky to get enough of in your diet.

Tip: Cucumbers are very low in calories and high in water and can keep you hydrated.

1 cup unsweetened vanilla almond milk
¼ cup pumpkin seeds
¼ cup avocado
1 cup frozen kale
1 small cucumber ¼ cup parsley
1 Medjool date, pitted
1 cup ice

In a blender, combine the milk and pumpkin seeds and process into a thick paste. Add remaining ingredients and blend until smooth. Serve right away.

<u>VARIATION</u>: Substitute the avocado with tofu.

Nutritional info: calories: 400, fat: 23 grams, carbs: 39 grams, fiber: 10 grams, protein: 15 grams

Day 3
Apple and Ginger

JOINT-SUPPORTING, HEART-HEALTHY and HIGH-FIBER

Prepare your body for restful sleep with a smoothie made of melatoninrich cherries and digestion-promoting ginger. The added slow-burning carbohydrates from the oats and the protein from the milk make this smoothie a tasty sleep-inducing nightcap.

Tip: Ginger root is good for digestion and acts as an anti-inflammatory.

1 cup unsweetened, protein-fortified almond milk
2 tablespoons ground flaxseed
1 medium apple, cored and chopped
¾ cup frozen cherries
1 tablespoon chopped ginger root
¼ cup rolled oats
1 cup ice

In a blender, combine the milk and flaxseed and process into a thick paste.

Add the remaining ingredients and blend until smooth. Serve right away.

Nutritional info: calories: 380, fat: 8 grams, carbs: 62 grams, fiber: 15 grams, protein: 11 grams

Day 4
Pineapple Turmeric Green Cleanser

JOINT-SUPPORTING and HIGH-FIBER

This cleansing smoothie is made from pineapple, which contains bromelain, a type of natural digestive enzyme, and the spices ginger and turmeric, powerful anti-inflammatories.

Tip: Psyllium husk is a soluble fiber than can lower cholesterol and ease symptoms of diarrhea and constipation.

½ cup raw cashews
1 cup unsweetened, protein-fortified almond milk
½ cup avocado
1 cup chopped fresh pineapple
1 cup frozen kale
½ cup frozen broccoli Juice of
½ lemon
1 tablespoon pysllium husk
1 tablespoon grated fresh ginger
¼ teaspoon ground turmeric
1 cup ice

In a blender, combine the cashews with the milk and process into a paste. Add remaining ingredients and blend until smooth. Serve right away.

<u>VARIATION</u>: Substitute the cashews with Brazil nuts.

Nutritional info: calories: 380, fat: 19 grams, carbs: 40 grams, fiber: 14 grams, protein: 14 grams.

Day 5
Green UP

HIGH-PROTEIN

This green smoothie is high in healthy omega-3 and monounsaturated fats, vitamins A and C, folate, and fiber. The mint will stimulate your digestion, while the high protein content will keep you feeling full and satisfied for hours.

Tip: Try freezing the avocado and tofu to make your smoothie extra thick.

1 cup silken tofu
2 tablespoons ground flaxseed
1 cup frozen kale
¼ cup avocado
½ frozen banana
1 tablespoon fresh mint
1 cup ice

In a blender, combine tofu, frozen kale, avocado and banana and blend until smooth. Add remaining ingredients and blend until smooth. Serve right away.

<u>VARIATION 1</u>: Substitute the tofu with soy yogurt.

<u>VARIATION 2</u>: Add a serving of protein powder.

Nutritional info: calories: 330, fat: 15 grams, carbs: 28 grams, fiber: 10 grams, protein: 16 grams

Day 6
Mango and Green Tea

BRAIN-BOOSTING

This smoothie will give you good clean energy that won't result in a crash. Rev up your metabolism with a smoothie made using antioxidant-rich green tea and stay satisfied for hours with plant-based hemp seed protein.

Tip: One cup of green tea has about 35mg of caffeine compared to 8 ounces of brewed coffee, which contains about 200mg of caffeine.

1 cup brewed and cooled green tea
1 (6-ounce) container of plain yogurt 1 cup frozen mango
1 cup frozen spinach
2 tablespoons hemp seeds
1 to 2 Medjool dates, pitted
1 cup ice

In a blender, combine frozen spinach, hemp seeds and green tea blend until smooth. Add remaining ingredients and blend until smooth. Serve right away.

<u>VARIATION 1</u>: Substitute yogurt or tofu for the almond milk.

<u>VARIATION 2</u>: Add ¼ cup rolled oats for additional slow-burning carbs.

Nutritional info: calories: 371, fat: 19 grams, carbs: 50 grams, fiber: 9 grams, protein: 7 grams

Day 7

Green Pear

BEAUTY-BOOSTING, HIGH-PROTEIN and HIGH-FIBER

Start your week on an energizing note with this green smoothie featuring skin-nourishing pears and plantbased protein. Pears are ranked as one of the most easily digested fruits and are also considered to be a low-allergy food. The skin of this fruit contains an array of phytochemicals and about half of the pear's fiber, so leave it on for maximum nutritional benefits.

Tip: Edamame contains phytoestrogens that can reduce the risk for chronic diseases and, when blended, lend a creamy consistency.

1 cup unsweetened vanilla almond milk
1 cup frozen kale
½ cup shelled edamame
1 medium pear, diced
2 tablespoons ground flaxseed
1 teaspoon grated fresh ginger
1 cup ice In a blender, combine all of the ingredients and blend until smooth. Serve right away.

In a blender, combine frozen kale , ginger and pear blend until smooth. Add remaining ingredients and blend until smooth. Serve right away.

Nutritional info: calories: 341, fat: 11 grams, carbs: 47 grams, fiber: 16 grams, protein: 16 grams

Day 8
Dandelion Green

HIGH-FIBER and PROTEIN-PACKED

The high-fiber, low-calorie jicama adds a pear-like flavor to this smoothie made with green fruits and vegetables. Both cleansing and hydrating, this smoothie will leave you feeling fueled and energized.

Tip: Dandelion greens are high in calcium and loaded with vitamins, minerals, and antioxidants. Because they have a bitter taste, they are best paired with a sweet fruit like bananas to mask their flavor.

1 (11-ounce) container coconut water
1 (6-ounce) container vanilla soy yogurt
1 cup frozen spinach
1 cup fresh dandelion greens
½ cup jicama
¼ cup avocado
½ frozen banana
1 tablespoon lime juice
1 cup ice

In a blender combine all the ingredients and blend until smooth. Serve right away.

<u>VARIATION</u>: Substitute cucumber for the jicama.

Nutritional info: calories: 417, fat: 9 grams, carbs: 76 grams, fiber: 15 grams, protein: 16 grams

Day 9
Green Goddess

BEAUTY-BOOSTING and HIGH-FIBER

This free radical–fighting smoothie will give you twice your daily recommended intake of vitamin C, omega-3 fats, and hydrating electrolytes. The kiwi gives this combination an invigorating taste reminiscent of strawberries and bananas.

Tip: Eating a couple of kiwifruit each day can lower your triglyceride levels and reduce your risk for blood clots.

1 (11-ounce) container coconut water
1 (6-ounce) container vanilla soy yogurt
1 cup frozen spinach
1 kiwi, peeled and sliced
2 tablespoons ground flaxseed

In a blender, combine vanilla soy yogurt, spinach, coconut water and blend until smooth. Add remaining ingredients and blend until smooth. Serve right away.

VARIATION 1: Substitute almond milk for the coconut water for a creamier smoothie.

VARIATION 2: Add an additional kiwi to boost the fiber and vitamin C content.

Nutritional info: calories: 377, fat: 9 grams, carbs: 64 grams, fiber: 13 grams, protein: 16 grams

Day 10
Pumpkin Seeds and Greens

LOW-CALORIE

This spicy, green smoothie has ingredients that will hydrate and fuel you, leaving you feeling calm and nourished. Pumpkin seeds are rich in magnesium, one of the most critical minerals for helping your body cope with stress, along with healthy fats, f iber, and minerals. Drink up some cool refreshment and just breathe.

Tip: Sprouting seeds, like pumpkin, multiply the nutritional profile. The germination process also makes them easier to digest and increases their enzyme content.

1 cup unsweetened vanilla almond milk
1 cup frozen kale
½ frozen banana
¼ cup pumpkin seeds
½ teaspoon grated ginger
1 cup ice

In a blender, combine kale, banana, pumpkin seeds and and blend until smooth. Add remaining ingredients and blend until smooth. Serve right away. Serve right away.

<u>VARIATION</u>: Substitute yogurt or tofu for the almond milk.

Nutritional info: calories: 260, fat: 15 grams, carbs: 23 grams, fiber: 5 grams, protein: 11 grams

Day 11
Pineapple and Spinach with Cilantro and Ginger

BEAUTY-BOOSTING and HIGH-FIBER

This frosty blend of spinach, pineapple and cilantro will taste refreshing and light. Fresh ginger seals the deal on this drink that's filled with herbaceous goodness.

Tip: Ginger has a long tradition of being effective in alleviating discomfort, pain in the stomach. It's regarded as an excellent carminative, this substance promote the elimination of excessive gas from the digestive system, and soothes the intestinal tract. Colic and dyspepsia respond particularly well to ginger.

1 ½ cups low-fat milk
1 cup frozen pineapple
½ cup chopped spinach
¼ cup chopped cilantro
½ tsp freshly grated ginger

In a blender combine pineapple, combine milk, spinach, cilantro, ginger, and black pepper to taste. Blend on high speed until smooth. Serve right away.

Nutritional info: calories: 126, fat: 2 grams, carbs: 17 grams, fiber: 1 grams, protein: 7 grams

Day 12

Roasted Grapes with Banana

JOINT-SUPPORTING

Grapes are berries, and roasting them brings their sweetness to another level. Use a combination of red - green grapes for an even more unexpected smoothie experience.

Tip: Eating more fiber from vegetables and fruits like bananas has repeatedly been linked to lower body weight and weight loss

2 cups halved grapes
1 frozen medium banana

Pre-heat the oven to 400°F. Place grapes on a baking pan and roast for 6 minutes. Remove the pan, transfer grapes to a bowl, and place the bowl in the freezer for 4 to 5 minutes.

In a blender, combine 1 cup water, cooled grapes, and banana. Blend high speed until smooth. Serve right away.

Nutritional info: calories: 228, fat: 1 grams, carbs: 44 grams, fiber: 5 grams, protein: 2 grams

Day 13
Spinach & Pearswith Lemon

BRAIN-BOOSTING

Pear and Spinach should seem like a no-brainer pairing. Pears bring filling fiber, while spinach offers vitamins and nutrients to keep you strong to the finish.

Tips: Spinach may be one of the healthiest foods on earth. It supplies large amounts of the eye-healthy carotenoids lutein and zeaxanthin, which have been shown to lower risk of cataract development. The folate, vitamin C, potassium, magnesium and antioxidant phytonutrients in spinach promote heart health.

1 cup milk skim
2 medium pears, Anjou or Bartlett varieties recommended, peeled, cored, and diced
2 cups raw baby spinach
1 tbsp freshly squeezed lemon juice

In a blender, combine milk, pears, spinach, lemon juice, and as many ice cubes as needed. Blend high speed until smooth. Serve right away.

Nutritional info: calories: 131, fat: 1 grams, carbs: 23 grams, fiber: 5 grams, protein: 5 grams

Day 14

Peachy Green tea with Ginger and Honey

PROTECTIVE POLYPHENOLS

Frozen peaches blend beautifully, and because they're as nutritious as fresh, no need for peeling! Brewed tea offers a boost of flavor (and antioxidants) for no added calories.

Tip: Ginger has been used to inflammatory conditions. It has also been found to positively aid people suffering from inflammation due to osteoarthritis.

1½ cups chilled brewed green tea
3 cups frozen peaches
1 cup nonfat Greek yogurt
1 tbsp honey
1 tsp freshly grated ginger

In a blender combine peaches, yogurt, combine green tea, honey, and ginger and blend high speed until smooth. Serve right away.

Nutritional info: calories: 153, fat: 0 grams, carbs: 38 grams, fiber: 3 grams, protein: 8 grams

Day 15
Sweet Pea Shakewith Pineapple and Lime

HIGH-PROTEIN

One of the best plant-based protein powders is made from peas. It has a mild flavor and blends beautifully, and most brands contain about 20 grams of protein per serving.

Tip: Pineapple could help shorten viral and bacterial infections and strengthen your bones.

2 cups unsweetened coconut milk beverage
½ cup frozen peas
1 cup frozen pineapple
2 ounces unsweetened pea protein powder
zest and juice of 1 lime

In a blender, combine peas, pineapple, coconut milk, protein powder, lime zest and juice. Blend high speed until smooth. Pour the mixture into two chilled glasses and serve.

Nutritional info: calories: 204, fat: 4 grams, carbs: 11 grams, fiber: 3 grams, protein: 22 grams

Day 16
Banana and Spinach with Green tea and Chia seeds

BEAUTY-BOOSTING

Kickstart your day with a jolt of caffeine and a few healthy calories? This green drink has the ideal balance of healthy protein carbs and fat.

Tip: Chia seeds are high in antioxidants that help protect the delicate fats in the seeds.

2 cups chilled brewed green tea
1 tbsp chia seeds
2 tbsp almond butter
1 frozen medium banana
1 cup baby spinach

In a blender, combine chia seeds, green tea, almond butter, banana, and spinach. Blend high speed until smooth. Pour the mixture into two chilled glasses and serve immediately.

Nutritional info: calories: 177, fat: 10 grams, carbs: 8 grams, fiber: 5 grams, protein: 6 grams

Day 17

Banana and Clementine with Wheatgrass and Coconut

LOW-CALORIE

Wheatgrass can be hard to find, but wheatgrass powder is another way to take antioxidant power. And a little goes a long way!

Tip: Wheatgrass might help:prevent diseases, reduce oxidative stress, boost the metabolism and storage of energy

1½ cups coconut water
1 frozen medium banana
1 clementine
2 tsp wheatgrass powder

In a blender, combine banana, clementine, coconut water and wheatgrass powder. Blend high speed until smooth. Pour the mixture into two glasses and serve immediately.

Nutritional info: calories: 111, fat: 0 grams, carbs: 17 grams, fiber: 3 grams, protein: 2 grams

Day 18
Banana with Matcha Milk and Honey

NATURAL DETOX

Matcha powder is finely ground green tea, giving you nutrients and inflammation-fighting antioxidants. Matcha to improved attention and memory.

Tip: Matcha milk contains L-Theanine, which is very calming and relaxing to the body.

1 cup unsweetened soy milk
½ cup chilled brewed green tea
2 tsp matcha powder
1 tbsp honey
1 frozen medium banana

In a blender, combine matcha, honey, soy milk, green tea and banana. Blend high speed until smooth.Pour the mixture into chilled glasse and serve.

Nutritional info: calories: 135, fat: 2 grams, carbs: 25 grams, fiber: 2 grams, protein: 4 grams

Day 19
Kale Lemonade with Honey

LOW-CALORIE

This low-calorie juice is a vitamin-filled complement to any meal–and without a lot of sugar. If you're not a fan of kale, its natural sweetness will pleasantly surprise you.

Tip: Kale is an excellent source of vitamin C, vitamin A, manganese and is a good source of dietary fiber, vitamin B6, copper, calcium and potassium.

juice of **2** lemons
1 cup chopped kale
1 tbsp honey

In a blender combine 2 cups water, kale, honey, lemon juice, and as 2 ice cubes as needed. Blend high speed until smooth. Pour the mixture into chilled glasse and serve.

Nutritional info: calories: 55, fat: 0 grams, carbs: 18 grams, fiber: 1 grams, protein: 2 grams

Day 20

Key Lime and Romaine with Banana and Coconut

LOW-FAT

Lettuce in a smoothie? Yeah! Romaine's mild freshness works beautifully with tangy key limes. Serve this smoothie over ice and start sipping your salad!

Tip: Romaine is a good source of Riboflavin, Magnesium, Vitamin B6, Calcium, Copper and Phosphorus.

2 cups coconut water
juice of **2** key limes
1 cup chopped romaine lettuce
1 frozen medium banana

In a blender, combine coconut water, key lime juice, romaine lettuce, and banana. Blend on high speed until smooth. Place ½ cup ice into two glasses, pour the mixture over the ice, and serve.

Nutritional info: calories: 123, fat: 0 grams, carbs: 16 grams, fiber: 5 grams, protein: 2 grams

Day 21
Cilantro and Avocado with a splash of Lime

BEAUTY-BOOSTING

This is a green drink for when you aren't in the mood for something sweet. Enjoy this creamy smoothie with a light lunch.

Tip: This herb can help calm the nerves and improve sleep quality due to its natural sedative properties.

2 cups coconut water
1 avocado
¼ cup fresh cilantro, leaves and stems
juice of ½ lime

In a blender, combine avocado, cilantro, coconut water and many ice cubes as needed. Blend on high speed until smooth. Pour the mixture into chilled glass and serve immediately.

Nutritional info: calories: 162, fat: 11 grams, carbs: 20 grams, fiber: 6 grams, protein: 2 grams

Day 22
Kombucha with Spinach

LOW-CALORIE

You'll be amazed at how refreshing this green drink is. Mix kombucha along with some spinach and blend with ice cubes for a frosty drink / blend and then pour over ice.

Tip: Raw kombucha is a good source of probiotics that may be beneficial for your digestive health

1½ cups kombucha
1 cup baby spinach

In a blender, combine baby spinach, kombucha and as many ice cubes as needed. Blend on high speed until smooth. Pour the mixture into chilled glasse and serve immediately.

Nutritional info: calories: 33, fat: 0 grams, carbs: 6 grams, fiber: 1 grams, protein: 1 grams

Day 23
Cucumber with Lime

NATURAL DETOX

Use an cucumber which have smaller seeds than regular cucumbers to maximize the nutrients in this drink. And leave the skin of cucumber for more minerals.

Tip: Cucumber also contains 19.9 milligrams (mg) of calcium. Adults need 1,000–1,200 mg of calcium a day, depending on sex and age.

1 cucumber, diced
zest and juice of 1 lime

In a blender, combine cucumber, 2 cups water, lime zest and juice, and as many ice cubes as needed. Blend on high speed until smooth. Pour the mixture into two chilled glasses and serve.

Nutritional info: calories: 43, fat: 0 grams, carbs: 4 grams, fiber: 3 grams, protein: 1 grams

Day 24
Kale and Green Apple with Ginger

SKIN DETOX

Choose Bio apples and leave the skin to gain all the fiber apples. You don't have to limit this smoothie to just green apples, use any type of apple whatever's in season.

Tip: Green apple contains Vitamin C, helps in preventing skin cells damage by free radicals and thus reduces the chances of skin cancer.

1½ cups unsweetened almond milk
2 cups chopped kale
2 medium green apples, cored and diced
1 tsp freshly grated ginger

In a blender combine almond kale, apples, milkginger and as many ice cubes as needed. Blend on high speed until smooth. Pour the mixture into chilled glasse and serve.

Nutritional info: calories: 140, fat: 2 grams, carbs: 41 grams, fiber: 8 grams, protein: 3 grams

Day 25
Tomatillo Whirl with Honey and Lime

LOW-FAT

There's more to tomatillos than making salsa! This tangy green drink is filling and offers many nutrients, like fiber, potassium, niacin, and iron–for about 40 calories per serving.

Tip: Fresh tomate is one of the vegetables that has the least sodium to potassium ratio.

2 tomatillos, husks removed and flesh roughly chopped
1 tbsp honey
juice of 1 lime

In a blender combine honey, lime juice, 11/4 cups water, tomatillos, as ice cubes as needed, sea salt to taste. Blend on high speed until smooth. Pour the mixture into chilled glasse and serve immediately.

Nutritional info: calories: 43, fat: 0 grams, carbs: 11 grams, fiber: 1 grams, protein: 0 grams

Day 26
Mango pops with Dates and Spinach

BRAIN-BOOSTING

Popsicles and breackfast, Who says you can't do both? These vitamin and fiber filled frozen treats are actually perfect for breakfast on a hot summer day.

Tip: Dates have been studied for their potential to promote and ease late-term labor in pregnant women.

1 cup unsweetened soy milk
1 cup frozen mango
2 pitted dates
1 cup baby spinach
½ cup granola

In a blender, combine soy milk, mango, dates, and spinach. Blend on high speed until smooth. Pour the mixture into four popsicle molds and stir a little granola into each mold. Freeze for at least 4 hours before serving.

Nutritional info: calories: 98, fat: 2 grams, carbs: 19 grams, fiber: 3 grams, protein: 5 grams

Day 27
Spinach and Bananas with Dates

POTASSIUM BOMB

Power up your day with this naturally sweetened green drink. This a great smoothie for those who want an introduction to a green drink–and this one has a lot of great flavor.

Tip: Ripen bananas at room temperature and add them to cereal for a tasty breakfast.

2 cups low-fat milk
2 medium bananas
2 large dates, pitted and chopped
1 cup baby spinach

In a blender, combine dates, spinach, milk, bananas, and as many ice cubes as needed. Blend on high speed until smooth. Pour the mixture into chilled glass and serve immediately.

Nutritional info: calories: 242, fat: 3 grams, carbs: 46 grams, fiber: 6 grams, protein: 11 grams

Day 28
Coconut and Banana with Avocado Bliss

BOOST HEART HEALTH

Nothing makes a green smoothie creamier than an avocado. Use an extra ripe banana for just the right level of sweetness. This simple blend is filled with heart healthy fats and fiber.

Tip: Avocados are very high in potassium.14% of the recommended daily allowance (RDA)

1½ cups unsweetened coconut milk beverage
1 avocado
1 frozen medium banana

In a blender, combine coconut milk, 1/2 cup water, avocado and banana. Blend on high speed until smooth. Pour the mixture into chilled glass and serve immediately.

Nutritional info: calories: 200, fat: 14 grams, carbs: 20 grams, fiber: 6 grams, protein: 2 grams

Day 29
Spinach and Apple with Broccoli and Banana
NATURAL DETOX

This smoothie will get your engine running with plenty of goodness from fruits and vegetables, including coconut water and banana teaming up for a potassium-loaded experience.

Tip: Sulforaphane and other natural compounds in broccoli might stop cancer cells from forming in your body.

1 cup coconut water
½ cup broccoli
½ cup baby spinach
1 green apple, cored and chopped
1 medium banana

In a blender, combine coconut water, spinach, broccoli, apple and banana. Blend on high speed until smooth. Pour the mixture into chilled glass and serve immediately.

Nutritional info: calories: 130, fat: 0 grams, carbs: 33 grams, fiber: 5 grams, protein: 2 grams

Day 30
Kiwi and Avocado with Mint

FRESH BREATH

A few delicious green ingredients blended with coconut milk make this a vitamin-filled smoothie. It's 25% of your daily fiber, sip on this to keep you satisfied for hours.

Tip: Peppermint oil contains menthol, which is thought to help alleviate IBS through its relaxing effects on the muscles of the digestive tract

1 cup unsweetened coconut milk
1 avocado
1 kiwi
2 tbsp chopped fresh mint leaves

In a blender, combine avocado, kiwi, coconut milk, mint and as many ice cubes as needed. Blend on high speed until smooth.Pour the mixture into two chilled glasses and serve immediately.

Nutritional info: calories: 157, fat: 13 grams, carbs: 11 grams, fiber: 6 grams, protein: 2 grams

Day 31
Parsley and Pineapple with spinach and banana

LOW-FAT

Stop thinking about parsley as a garnish. It's actually a nutrient powerhouse. This herb boasts vitamins A, C, and K as well as minerals, like potassium, iron, and calcium.

Tip: Along with eating a balanced diet, adding parsley to your cooking may help support healthy blood sugar levels.

2¼ cups coconut water
2 cups frozen pineapple
¼ cup roughly chopped parsley
2 cups baby spinach
1 medium frozen banana

In a blender, combine pineapple, coconut water, parsley, spinach, and banana. Blend on high speed until smooth. Pour the mixture into two chilled glasses and serve immediately.

Nutritional info: calories: 178, fat: 1 grams, carbs: 44 grams, fiber: 4 grams, protein: 3 grams

Day 32

Ginger Detox with Pineapple

DETOX DAY

Detox the natural way with this blend of tummy pleasing ginger and inflammation fighting pineapple. This combo will also help promote a glowing complexion.

Tip: Ginger can be used fresh, dried, powdered, or as an oil or juice, and is sometimes added to processed foods and cosmetics.

1½ cups unsweetened almond milk
juice of **1** lemon
1½ cups frozen pineapple
2 tsp freshly grated ginger

In a blender, combine lemon juice, almond milk, pineapple and ginger. Blend on high speed until smooth. Pour the mixture into chilled glass and serve immediately.

Nutritional info: calories: 97, fat: 3 grams, carbs: 18 grams, fiber: 3 grams, protein: 2 grams

Day 33
Zucchini Blast with Bok Choy and Lemon

LOW-CALORIE

This is a burst of green goodness to help curb cravings between meals. Bok choy is a Chinese cabbage that in this smoothie provides just the right amount of bite.

Tip: Studies have shown that some people who eat more cruciferous vegetables have a lower risk of developing lung, prostate, and colon cancer.

½ zucchini
1 small baby bok choy, trimmed roughly chopped
juice of **1** lemon

In a blender, combine 1 cup water, lemon juice, zucchini, bok choy and ice cubes as needed. Blend on high speed until smooth. Pour the mixture into glass and serve immediately.

Nutritional info: calories: 17, fat: 0 grams, carbs: 4 grams, fiber: 1 grams, protein: 1 grams

Day 34
Lemon with Kale Chiller

HIGH-PROTEIN

Coconut flavored Greek yogurt and protein powder team up with kale and lemon for a green smoothie that's ideal for any healthconscious sipper. It will tempt all your taste buds.

Tip: The fiber, potassium, vitamin C and vitamin B6 found in kale all support heart health.

1 cup chopped kale
1 cup coconut greek yogurt
1 scoop protein powder
juice of **1** lemon

In a blender, combine kale, 11/2 cups water, yogurt, protein powder, and lemon zest and juice. Blend on high speed until smooth. Pour the mixture into chilled glass and serve.

Nutritional info: calories: 148, fat: 4 grams, carbs: 14 grams, fiber: 1 grams, protein: 15 grams

Day 35
Power Green Smoothie

HIGH-POWER

This is the ultimate greens-based smoothie. You can vary the greens and the ratio used, adding less kale and more spinach if you like or throwing in some additional collards.

Tip: The vitamin K in mustard greens is essential for good health. Vitamin "K" is a fat soluble vitamin and helps with blood clotting functions in the body.

¼ cup green kale
¼ cup collard greens
¼ cup fresh baby spinach
¼ cup mustard greens
¼ cup frozen unsweetened pineapple, chopped
¼ cup sliced fresh or frozen strawberries
¼ medium banana, sliced
¼ cup almond milk

In a blender combine green kale, spinach, mustard, banana and blend on high speed until smooth. Add remaining ingredients and blend until smooth. Serve immediately.

Nutritional info: calories: 292, fat: 2 grams, carbs: 28 grams, fiber: 4 grams, protein: 2 grams

Day 36
Spinach and Agave nectar

FRUCTOSE BOMB

Spinach, banana, and kiwi fruit give a healthy vitamin and antioxidant rich boost to your day as key ingredients in this very tasty smoothie.

Tip: Agave nectar has a low GI primarily because almost all of the sugar in it is fructose. It has very little glucose, at least when compared to regular sugar.

¼ cup plain 2% reduced fat Greek yogurt
1¼ cups fresh baby spinach
½ cups plain sweetened almond milk
¼ tablespoon agave nectar or honey
½ frozen medium bananas, sliced
½ chopped peeled kiwifruit

In a blender place the yogurt add the spinach, almond milk, bananas, agave nectar and kiwifruit and blend on high speed until smooth. Serve.

Nutritional info: calories: 161, fat: 3 grams, carbs: 30 grams, fiber: 4 grams, protein: 7 grams

Day 37
Avocado and fresh Lime Juice

GOOD FATS

Avocado adds loads of nutrients to this cool, refreshing vietnamese specialty. The monounsaturated fats and fiber found in avocado help lower cholesterol while keeping you full longer. It's best served icy cold, straight from the blender.

Tip: *Over 75% of the fats in avocados is unsaturated fat, monounsaturated and polyunsaturated fat. That fats don't raise LDL levels (the unhealthy type of cholesterol) which is helpful for a healthy heart.*

¼ ripe avocado
½ cups sweetened almond milk
¼ cup crushed ice
¼ cup fat free sweetened condensed milk
½ tablespoons fresh lime juice
¼ tablespoon chopped slivered almonds, toasted

Cut the avocado in half lengthwise. Scoop the pulp from the avocado halves into a blender. Add the almond milk , avocado, condensed milk and fresh lime juice; process until smooth. Top each serving with toasted almonds and serve.

Nutritional info: calories: 142, fat: 7 grams, carbs: 17 grams, fiber: 3 grams, protein: 3 grams

Day 38
Melon with Spinach and Kiwi

HIGH-PROTEIN

Try this recipe in the summer when honeydew melon is at its peak. You can garnish the glasses with wheels of additional peeled, sliced kiwifruit.

Tip: Melons are high in fiber, Vitamin C, potassium, and a few B vitamins like B6. Cantaloupe melons are considered very nutrient-dense because of their high Vitamin A content. One cup on cantaloupe contains 120% RDA of Vitamin A.

½ cup vanilla light soy milk
½ container fat free Greek yogurt with honey
½ cubed peeled kiwifruit
½ cup cubed honeydew melon
½ cup fresh baby spinach
½ cup sliced banana, frozen

In a blender, combine soy milk, greek yogurt, kiwi, spinach and blend until smooth. Add remaining ingredients and blend until smooth. Pour the mixture into chilled glass and serve.

Nutritional info: calories: 225, fat: 1 grams, carbs: 48 grams, fiber: 4 grams, protein: 10 grams

Day 39
Cucumber with Apple and Mint

SKIN CARE

This is the perfect blend of fruit and vegetables that has been lightly—and naturally—sweetened and whirred into a refreshing drink. This smoothie offers a half-cup of vegetables, plus a little fruit. It's ideal as a snack or healthy breakfast. To dress it up, garnish with thin cucumber slices.

Tip: Applying sliced cucumber directly to the skin can help cool and soothe the skin and reduce swelling and irritation. It can alleviate sunburn. Placed on the eyes, they can help decrease morning puffiness.

½ cup chopped seeded peeled cucumber (about ½ pound)
½ cup frozen 100% apple juice concentrate
¼ cup cold water
¼ cup chopped fresh mint
5 ice cubes

Place all the ingredients in a blender. Process 2 minutes or until smooth. Pour the mixture into chilled glass and serve.

Nutritional info: calories: 91, fat: 0,5 grams, carbs: 22 grams, fiber: 1 grams, protein: 1 grams

Day 40
Cucumber lightweight smoothie

LOW-FAT

Yogurt drinks are popular in the Middle East and South Asia. We like ours with pureed cucumber, herbs and a spritz of club soda. If the cucumber peels and seeds are tender, they don't need to be removed.

Tip: One lemon provides about 30 mg of vitamin C, which is 51% of the reference daily intake RDA

½ cups cold plain fat free yogurt
½ cups chopped cold cucumbers, plus 4 slices
½ tablespoons packed coarsely chopped fresh dill
½ tablespoons packed coarsely chopped fresh basil
½ tablespoons packed coarsely chopped fresh mint leaves
½ tablespoons fresh lemon juice
3 ice cubes
¼ teaspoon fine sea salt
¼ cups cold club soda or sparkling water

Place the yogurt, chopped cucumbers, herbs, lemon juice, 3 ice cubes, and the salt in a blender. Pour the cucumber puree into glass. Fill the glasses with soda and stir. Add more ice if you like, and garnish with cucumber slices.

Nutritional info: calories: 78, fat: 0,15 grams, carbs: 13 grams, fiber: 1 grams, protein: 7 grams

Day 41

Creamy Mango with Avocado and Lime

ANTI-AGE SMOOTHIE

These Mexican-grown mango are sweeter and more tender than many of the most common and widely available varieties. Look for them in the grocery store from late February to early August.

Tip: Mango is packed with polyphenols — plant compounds that function as antioxidants. It has a dozen different types: mangiferin, catechins, anthocyanins, quercetin, kaempferol, rhamnetin, benzoic acid and more.

¼ cup sliced ripe avocado
1 cup sliced Champagne mango
1 tablespoon fresh lime juice
1 tablespoon fresh mint
1 teaspoon honey
2 cups crushed ice

In a blender combine avocado, mango, lime juice, mint, honey process until smooth. Add crushed ice. Garnish with mint sprig, if desired. Pour the mixture into chilled glass and serve.

Nutritional info: calories: 185, fat: 6 grams, carbs: 35 grams, fiber: 5 grams, protein: 2 grams

Day 42
Spring Salad Smoothie with Cilantro

NATURAL DETOX

This cilantro-spiked smoothie is a tasty and untraditional way to get your greens.

Tip: Arsenic, aluminum, cadmium, lead and mercury can become resident in our body. This can lead to heart disease, neurological conditions, hormonal imbalances, infertility and much more. Cilantro, known scientifically as "Coriandrum sativum," has been shown to bind these toxic metals, loosening them from your body.

½ cup carrot juice
¼ cup chopped ripe avocado
¼ cup fresh baby spinach or mâche
¼ cup ice
3 tablespoons frozen wheatgrass juice
2 tablespoons chopped fresh cilantro
1½ tablespoons fresh lemon juice
1 tablespoon ground flaxseed
½ teaspoon matcha tea powder
Pinch of fine sea salt

Place all the ingredients in a blender. Blend on high speed until smooth add more ice if you like and serve immediately.

Nutritional info: calories: 173, fat: 8 grams, carbs: 20 grams, fiber: 6 grams, protein: 7 grams

Day 43
Tropical Treat Smoothie

HIGH POWER

The lime juice and fresh mint give this drink a bright, fresh flavor.

Tip: Research has linked the anti-bacterial compounds in mint's essential oils (carvone and limonene) to helping reduce risk of potentially harmful bacteria, both the type found in affected food, and within your GI tract.

1 cup frozen unsweetened pineapple cubes
1 tablespoon fresh lime juice
1 tablespoon chopped fresh mint leaves
½ cup silken tofu
½ cup coconut sorbet
½ teaspoon minced peeled fresh ginger
2 tablespoons cold water

Place all the ingredients in a blender. Blend on high speed until smooth. Pour the mixture into chilled glass and garnish with pineapple wedge. Serve immediately.

Nutritional info: calories: 321, fat: 10 grams, carbs: 51 grams, fiber: 3 grams, protein: 8 grams

Day 44

Green Grape Bowl

CANDY GRAPE

In this smoothie bowl, green grapes add beautiful color and juicy freshness to a spinach-based smoothie. The juice from the grapes acts as your liquid here—you may need a little almond milk too—to blend this to a just-right consistency. You can also top this bowl with fresh pineapple or coconut flakes.

Tip: Grapes are sweet, very low-fat and relatively low calorie fruit. If you are trying reduce your processed food, grapes can be a good substitute for other goodies like candy, cookies or treats.

½ cup green grapes
½ cup fresh baby spinach
½ cup frozen unsweetened pineapple
½ frozen medium banana
Splash of plain unsweetened almond milk
Toppings:
½ banana, sliced
1 teaspoon chia seeds
1 tablespoon yogurt chips

Place the first 4 smoothie ingredients in a blender; process until smooth. If the mixture is thick add a almond milk until well combined. Pour into a bowl, and top with the chia seeds, banana sliced and yogurt chips.

Nutritional info: calories: 283, fat: 4 grams, carbs: 62 grams, fiber: 7 grams, protein: 4 grams

Day 45
Green Tea with Kiwi and Mango

ANTI AGE

Make a colorful and healthy smoothie pureeing mango, kiwifruit, and spinach with yogurt and honey and spooning into glasses in two layers.

Tip: Green tea is about 30% polyphenols by weight, including catechin called EGCG. Catechins are natural antioxidants, that help prevent cell damage.

1½ cups frozen cubed mango
¾ cup vanilla fat free yogurt, divided
¼ cup honey, divided
2 tablespoons water
½ teaspoon lime zest
1 quartered and peeled kiwifruit
1 cups ice cubes
½ cup packed fresh baby spinach
1 tablespoons bottled green tea

Place the mango, ¼ cup of the yogurt, ¼ tablespoons of the honey, ½ tablespoons water, and lime zest in a blender; process until smooth, stirring occasionally. Place the glasses in the freezer. Rinse the blender container. Place the remaining ingredients in the blender; process until smooth, stirring occasionally. Gently spoon the green tea–kiwifruit mixture onto the mango mixture.

Nutritional info: calories: 204, fat: 1 grams, carbs: 52 grams, fiber: 2 grams, protein: 3 grams

Day 46

Grape fruit with Fennel and Avocado

HEART HEALTH

Avocado, grapefruit, and fennel are a popular salad trio; here's a drinkable version. Skewer extra apple and avocado slices for a pretty garnish, if desired.

Tip: The fiber, potassium, folate, vitamin C, vitamin B-6, and phytonutrient content in fennel, coupled with its lack of cholesterol, all support heart health.

½ cups fresh grapefruit juice (5 grapefruit)
½ cups chopped fennel
½ cups (½-inch) chunks peeled Gala apple
¼ cup diced ripe avocado (1 small)
¾ tablespoons honey
½ tablespoons chopped fennel fronds

In a blender, grapefruit juice, fennel, honey, apple and blend until smooth. Add remaining ingredients and blend until smooth. Pour the mixture into chilled glass and serve.

Nutritional info: calories: 162, fat: 4 grams, carbs: 34 grams, fiber: 7 grams, protein: 2 grams

Day 47
Spiced Green Tea

SKIN CARE

Green tea has been shown to have a host of health-promoting properties, including lowering cholesterol and improving blood flow. To make strong tea for this smoothie, brew 1 green tea bags in 3 ounces of boiling water and refrigerate.

Tip: Pears contain various compounds that may exhibit anticancer properties. Their cinnamic acid and anthocyanin contents have been shown to fight cancer.

½ cup strong green tea, chilled
bit teaspoon cayenne pepper
Juice of **1** lemon
1 teaspoons agave nectar
½ pear, skin on, cut into pieces
2 tablespoons plain fat-free yogurt
3 ice cubes

In a blender combine green tea, pepper, lemon and blend. Add remaining ingredients and blend until smooth. Serve immediately.

Nutritional info: calories: 73, fat: 0.2 grams, carbs: 19 grams, fiber: 2 grams, protein: 1 grams

Day 48
Cocoa Peanut

HIGH-PROTEIN

This smoothie with Spinach is a nutritional powerhouse that tastes like a liquid peanut butter cup, t's the perfect breakfast recipe and a great way to start any day!

Tip: Approximately 35% of peanut butter's total weight is from protein, making it one of the better sources of non-meat protein.

1½ cup almond milk
2½ tablespoons chocolate protein powder
½ tablespoons unsweetened cocoa powder
1 tablespoons peanut butter
½ banana
4 cup frozen spinach

In a blender combine almond milk, banana, spinach, peanut butter and blend. Add remaining ingredients and blend until smooth. Serve immediately.

Nutritional info: calories: 309, fat: 8 grams, carbs: 42 grams, fiber: 12 grams, protein: 29 grams

Day 49
Orange Bomb

HIGH-POWER

Orange Bomb is the perfect healthy breakfast or snack. It's a plant-based, clean eating smoothie recipe that is packed with grapefruit, oranges, greens and protein.

Tip: The antioxidant vitamin "C", when eaten in its natural form or applied topically, help to fight skin damage caused by the pollution, reduce wrinkles and improve overall skin texture. Vitamin C plays a vital role in the formation of collagen, the support system of your skin.

1½ cup unsweetened vanilla almond milk
½ big grapefruit (peeled)
1 medium orange (peeled)
1 frozen banana
1 cup frozen strawberries
2 cups frozen spinach
1 tablespoons honey

In a blender combine almond milk, banana, spinach, orange and blend. Add remaining ingredients and blend until smooth. Serve immediately.

Nutritional info: calories: 258, fat: 4 grams, carbs: 48 grams, fiber: 10 grams, protein: 14 grams

Day 50
Aloe Vera Smoothie

HIGH-DETOX

This Aloe Vera Smoothie packs in all the benefits of the superfood aloe plant in one healthy drink. It can help you boost your immunity and hydrate your skin.

Tip: The juice of the aloe vera plant has been used in particular as a skin soother. The viscous gel that oozes out of the leaves of this plant can cool minor burns or irritation and moisturize your skin.

½ cup filleted aloe vera gel
1 banana
½ cup kiwi
¼ cup ice
1½ cup coconut milk

In a blender combine coconut milk, banana, aloe vera gel, kiwi and blend. Add remaining ingredients and blend until smooth. Serve immediately.

Nutritional info: calories: 99, fat: 3 grams, carbs: 18 grams, fiber: 2 grams, protein: 2 grams

TROUBLESHOOTING GUIDE

Whenever you explore something new, there is a learning curve and a bit of experimentation involved. Don't get discouraged if your first smoothie turn out less than perfect. Smoothie making isn't difficult. However, each blender is different, so you might have to tweak the recipes as you get to know your machine. The most important thing to remember is to have fun and enjoy experimenting. You know what they say: practice makes perfect!

My smoothie is too chunky or grainy
Solution: There could be several things at work here. First, you might not have blended long enough. Blenders vary greatly in their power, so it just might be that your blender isn't cutting it (literally), and you need to let it run for a bit longer to fully break down the ingredients. Some blenders simply can't handle raw veggies and fruits, in which case you might consider using a food processor to grind the fruits, veggies, and nuts before adding them to your smoothie. Another cause could be that you need to add a bit more liquid. Try adding an additional ¼ cup of your milk of choice and blend. You may need to repeat this a few times. Lastly, filling your blender jar to high might result in less than ideal blending, especially if you have an older or low-powered blender. Try blending your liquid, base, fresh fruit, and

greens first, then add frozen fruit or ice and blend until smooth.

My smoothie is too thin

Solution: There are some ways to turn a watery smoothie into one that is thick and creamy. Try adding more frozen fruit, especially bananas, which can serve double duty by fixing the consistency, while masking any flavor snafus. If you have a high powered blender, you can also try freezing a portion of your liquid ingredients in ice cube trays. Almond milk, coffee, and even yogurt can be frozen and added directly to the blender.

My smoothie is too thick

Solution: To make your smoothie less thick without watering down the taste, add a bit more milk, half cup at a time until you get the desired consistency. You can also add more water, but doing so may water down the taste. Another thing is to remember to load your blender container by putting the liquids in first, then soft fruits or vegetables, greens, and frozen fruits or vegetables and ice on top.

My smoothie is too bitter

Solution: You accidently added arugula instead of spinach to your smoothie, and the result is a bitter-tasting drink. The best fix for a situation like this is to add banana, which in addition to being sweet, seems to neutralize bitter flavors. Pineapples and oranges both add lots of fruity sweetness, and strawberries are an especially good choice for green smoothies. Also try adding a bit of vanilla bean or vanilla extract, unsweetened cacao, or unsweetened cocoa powder. Keep a few plastic bags of frozen bananas and mango chunks on hand while you are testing different combinations. Another thing to remember is that baby greens are generally milder than mature greens. Also, your tastes change and adapt to new eating habits. Try working up to bitter greens by combining small amounts of them with spinach in your smoothie.

My smoothie is too sweet

Solution: Fruits contribute their own natural sweetness so it shouldn't be necessary to add other sweeteners like honey or agave. But if you find your smoothie tastes too sugary or too syrupy, try adding just a touch of fresh lemon juice to cut down on the sweetness.

My smoothie isn't sweet enough

Solution: There are a number of ways to naturally sweeten a smoothie without adding sugar. By far the mother of all smoothie sweeteners is the Medjool date. Not just any date, this "king of dates" is super sweet and has a caramel-like taste that is compatible with just about any smoothie recipe. If you have a high-speed blender, just remove the pit and toss the date in. For low-powered blenders, try f inely chopping it and soaking it in a little warm water before adding it to the liquid called for in the recipe. Blend it into a loose date paste before adding the rest of the smoothie ingredients. Another great sweetening method is to use overripe bananas. Simply peel, cut, and freeze them in bags, and then pop them into the blender for added sweetness, as a thickener, and to mask bitter flavors.

My smoothie isn't creamy enough
Solution: If your smoothie is lacking in the creaminess department, it may be that you need to adjust your liquid and solid ingredients to achieve the right texture. Some of the most magical sources of creaminess for smoothie heaven are nuts, nut butters, avocados, oatmeal (cooked or dry), cooked grains, nondairy yogurt, frozen bananas, and spinach.

My smoothie is chalky tasting
Solution: If you decide to try out some protein powders in your smoothie, beware that powders are a tricky business, varying greatly in terms of ingredient quality, taste, and texture. Some powders add a chalky or grainy texture, while others add a bit of creaminess. You may want to start with half of the recommended amount and add a bit more liquid to absorb the powder until you get the consistency that works for you.

CONCLUSION

I am hoping that this e-book put up has spoken back your question of "How to lose 25 pounds in 50 days?"

I realize dieting can be hard, specifically for the reason that all of your existence you were taught to get your nourishment simplest from real plated foods.

But green smoothies are changing the food regime with their high nutritional/Health benefit to our body system.

Being highly nutritious, safe, and powerful in weight loss in a very effective and efficient manner.

I will strongly vouch for the benefits of taking and drinking of those green smoothies mentioned in this e-book recipe.

Many have tried these recipes and witness tremendous changes in their body, transforming them within 50 days of trial.

www.ingramcontent.com/pod-product-compliance
Lightning Source LLC
Chambersburg PA
CBHW070835250726

48662CB00003B/1240